Psychiatric Principles and Applications for General Patient Care

Fourth Edition

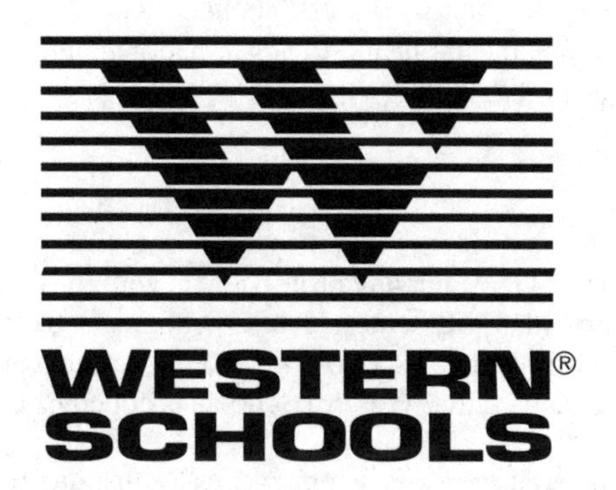

By

Bonnie Fossett, MSEd, RN, CS

and

Marlene Nadler-Moodie, MSN, RN, CS

Revised By:

Marshelle Thobaben, RN, MS, PHN, APNP, FNP

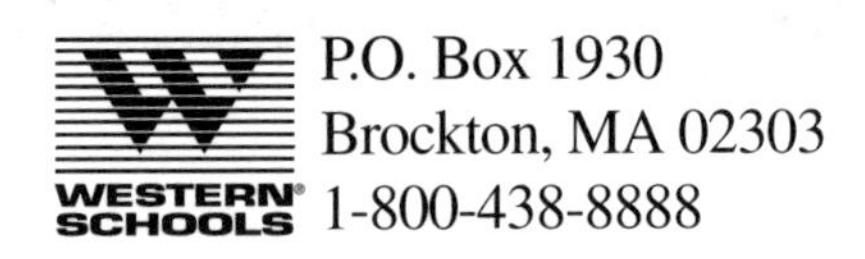
P.O. Box 1930
Brockton, MA 02303
1-800-438-8888

This book was previously titled: ***Psychiatric Aspects of General Patient Care***

ABOUT THE REVISING AUTHOR

Marshelle Thobaben, RN, MS, PHN, APNP, FNP, is chair and director of the Department of Nursing at Humboldt State University (HSU) in Arcata, CA. She has been a professor of nursing for nearly 30 years. She has published over 100 articles on psychosocial issues affecting clients and nurses in leading nursing journals and textbooks. Marshelle has presented at international and national conferences on issues affecting faculty, nurses, and clients, and has been nationally recognized for her work in elder abuse prevention and as one of the first nurses to develop a psychiatric nursing home health program. She is a consultant on legal cases involving abuse as well as on program development and psychiatric care in home health agencies. HSU has honored her as a Scholar of the Year for her outstanding research, creative activities, and publications.

Marshelle Thobaben has disclosed that she has no significant financial or other conflicts of interest pertaining to this course book.

ORIGINATING AUTHORS

Bonnie Fossett, MSEd, RN

Marlene Nadler-Moodie, MSN, APRN, BC, CNS, is currently the Clinical Nurse Specialist for Scripps Mercy Hospital in San Diego, CA; Adjunct Faculty for National University and a Psychiatric Hospital Surveyor for CMS. Ms. Nadler-Moodie has worked in the field of Psychiatric-Mental Health Nursing for more than 30 years, at least 25 as an Advanced Practice Nurse. She is Board Certified as a Clinical Nurse Specialist through American Nurses Credentialing Center. Ms. Nadler-Moodie has worked in many settings including inpatient acute care psychiatry and consultation-liaison, outpatient, home care, quality assurance and staff development as well as education. Ms. Nadler-Moodie is an active member of the American Psychiatric Nurses Association, serving as President of the California Chapter. She has been honored with the San Diego Psychiatric Mental Health Nurse of the Year Award and is listed in Who's Who in American Nursing. In addition she received the Outstanding Instructor Award at University of California, San Diego and several service awards for her professional commitments.

ABOUT THE SUBJECT MATTER REVIEWER

Jeanne B. Kozlak, MSN, CNS, APRN, BC, is a professor of psychiatric-mental health nursing at Humboldt State University in Arcata, CA. She has been a psychiatric nurse educator for 28 years and a psychiatric nurse consultant to various mental health and geriatric clinical facilities in northern California for the past 20 years. Professor Kozlak has provided expert witness consultation to attorneys in northern and southern California, and she now serves as part-time Patient's Rights Advocate for the mentally ill in Humboldt County (northern California). She has published work about psychiatric-mental health nursing in professional nursing journals and presented invited papers on various mental health topics at national and international conferences. Professor Kozlak is also an accomplished textbook and manuscript reviewer.

Copy Editor: Julie Munden
Indexer: Sylvia Coates

ISBN: 978-1-57801-111-7

 P0207SH

IMPORTANT: Read these instructions *BEFORE* proceeding!

Enclosed with your course book, you will find the FasTrax® answer sheet. Use this form to answer all the final exam questions that appear in this course book. If you are completing more than one course, be sure to write your answers on the appropriate answer sheet. Full instructions and complete grading details are printed on the FasTrax instruction sheet, also enclosed with your order. Please review them before starting. *If you are mailing your answer sheet(s) to Western Schools, we recommend you make a copy as a backup.*

ABOUT THIS COURSE

A Pretest is provided with each course to test your current knowledge base regarding the subject matter contained within this course. Your Final Exam is a multiple choice examination. **You will find the exam questions at the end of each chapter.**

In the event the course has less than 100 questions, mark your answers to the questions in the course book and leave the remaining answer boxes on the FasTrax answer sheet blank. **Use a black pen to fill in your answer sheet.**

A PASSING SCORE

You must score 70% or better in order to pass this course and receive your Certificate of Completion. Should you fail to achieve the required score, we will send you an additional FasTrax answer sheet so that you may make a second attempt to pass the course. Western Schools will allow you three chances to pass the same course...*at no extra charge!* After three failed attempts to pass the same course, your file will be closed.

RECORDING YOUR HOURS

Please monitor the time it takes to complete this course using the handy log sheet on the other side of this page. See below for transferring study hours to the course evaluation.

COURSE EVALUATIONS

In this course book, you will find a short evaluation about the course you are soon to complete. This information is vital to providing Western Schools with feedback on this course. The course evaluation answer section is in the lower right hand corner of the FasTrax answer sheet marked "Evaluation," with answers marked 1–23. Your answers are important to us; please take a few minutes to complete the evaluation.

On the back of the FasTrax instruction sheet, there is additional space to make any comments about the course, the school, and suggested new curriculum. Please mail the FasTrax instruction sheet, with your comments, back to Western Schools in the envelope provided with your course order.

TRANSFERRING STUDY TIME

Upon completion of the course, transfer the total study time from your log sheet to question 23 in the course evaluation. The answers will be in ranges; please choose the proper hour range that best represents your study time. You **MUST** log your study time under question 23 on the course evaluation.

EXTENSIONS

You have two (2) years from the date of enrollment to complete this course. A six (6) month extension may be purchased. If after 30 months from the original enrollment date you do not complete the course, *your file will be closed and no certificate can be issued.*

CHANGE OF ADDRESS?

In the event you have moved during the completion of this course, please call our student services department at 1-800-618-1670, and we will update your file.

A GUARANTEE TO WHICH YOU'LL GIVE HIGH HONORS

If any continuing education course fails to meet your expectations or if you are not satisfied in any manner, for any reason, you may return it for an exchange or a refund (less shipping and handling) within 30 days. Software, video, and audio courses must be returned unopened.

Thank you for enrolling at Western Schools!

WESTERN SCHOOLS
P.O. Box 1930
Brockton, MA 02303
(800) 438-8888
www.westernschools.com

Psychiatric Principles and Applications for General Patient Care

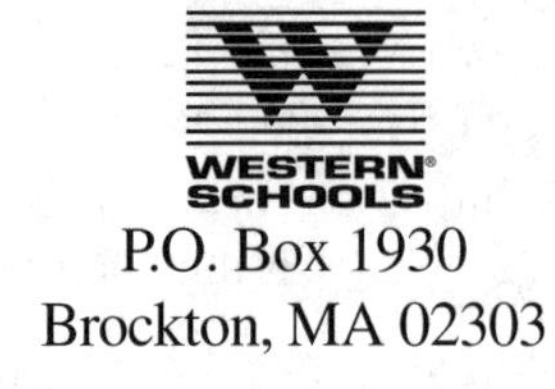

P.O. Box 1930
Brockton, MA 02303

Please use this log to total the number of hours you spend reading the text and taking the final examination (use 50-min hours).

Date	Hours Spent
____________	____________
____________	____________
____________	____________
____________	____________
____________	____________
____________	____________
____________	____________
____________	____________
____________	____________
____________	____________
____________	____________
____________	____________
____________	____________
____________	____________
TOTAL	

Please log your study hours with submission of your final exam. To log your study time, fill in the appropriate circle under question 23 of the FasTrax® answer sheet under the "Evaluation" section.

Psychiatric Principles and Applications for General Patient Care

WESTERN SCHOOLS
CONTINUING EDUCATION EVALUATION

Instructions: Mark your answers to the following questions with a black pen on the "Evaluation" section of your FasTrax® answer sheet provided with this course. You should not return this sheet. Please use the scale below to rate how well the course content met the educational objectives.

A	**Agree Strongly**	**C**	**Disagree Somewhat**
B	**Agree Somewhat**	**D**	**Disagree Strongly**

The course met the following education objectives:

1. Recognized major components of the communication process and identified interpersonal skills that are used to ensure good nursing care.
2. Demonstrated a psychosocial assessment and a mental status examination for patients.
3. Described the concept of anxiety, and how it relates to caring for patients who are experiencing anxiety.
4. Identified mood disorders and discussed how the principles of psychiatric nursing are used in the care of a patient with mood disorders.
5. Assessed a patient for suicidal ideation and specified nursing interventions that may be beneficial in caring for such a patient.
6. Recognized psychosis in a patient and appropriate interventions.
7. Identified substance-related disorders and discussed nursing interventions that may be useful in caring for a patient with a disorder of this type.
8. Explained the signs and symptoms of confusion in a patient and demonstrated how to apply sound principles of nursing care to confused patients.
9. Distinguished the manifestations of eating disorders, such as anorexia nervosa and bulimia nervosa, and appropriate intervention.
10. Described patients who are potentially aggressive and how to apply nursing interventions that can be used to prevent workplace violence.
11. Observed the major risk factors for noncompliance by patients and specified interventions to increase compliance.
12. Identified manipulative behaviors by patients and appropriate intervention.
13. Assessed common psychological responses to acute cardiac illness and those that occur in recovery phases.
14. Listed the classifications of psychotropic medications and indicated the applicable nursing interventions for administrating these drugs.
15. Described ethical and legal concerns in the practice of nursing when dealing with patients with psychiatric and mental health problems.

16. Identified the signs and symptoms of sleep disorders and be able to apply sound principles of nursing care to patients experiencing sleep disorders.

17. The content of this course was relevant to the objectives.

18. This offering met my professional education needs.

19. The objectives met the overall purpose/goal of the course.

20. The course was generally well-written and the subject matter explained thoroughly. (If no, please explain on the back of the FasTrax instruction sheet.)

21. The content of this course was appropriate for home study.

22. The final examination was well-written and at an appropriate level for the content of the course.

23. **PLEASE LOG YOUR STUDY HOURS WITH SUBMISSION OF YOUR FINAL EXAM.**
    Please choose which best represents the total study hours it took to complete this 30-hour course.

    A. Less than 25 hours
    B. 25–28 hours
    C. 29–32 hours
    D. Greater than 32 hours

CONTENTS

FIGURES AND TABLES

PRETEST

1. Begin this course by taking the pretest. Circle the answers to the questions on this page or write the answers on a separate sheet of paper. Do not log answers to the pretest questions on the FasTrax test sheet included with the course.
2. Compare your answers to the PRETEST KEY located in the back of the book. The pretest answer key indicates the course chapter where the content of that question is discussed. Make note of the questions you missed, so that you can focus on those areas as you complete the course.
3. Complete the course by reading each chapter and completing the exam questions at the end of the chapter. Answers to these exam questions should be logged on the FasTrax test sheet included with the course.

1. An example of support and reassurance, that ensures open communication between a nurse and patient is
   a. "I don't understand."
   b. "Go on."
   c. "How frustrating for you."
   d. "What you are thinking about?"

2. An example of a challenging phrase that closes communication between a nurse and patient is
   a. "That's wrong."
   b. "You can't be upset about that?"
   c. "It must be this way."
   d. "You can't be seeing pink elephants."

3. A nursing strategy for assessing psychosocial problems is
   a. establishing a therapeutic relationship with the patient.
   b. looking the psychiatric diagnosis up in the *DSM-IV-TR*.
   c. looking up the North American Nursing Diagnosis Association nursing diagnosis.
   d. reviewing your findings with your supervisor.

4. When a patient is experiencing mild anxiety, he or she has
   a. disorganized perceptions.
   b. misperceptions of stimuli.
   c. difficulty concentrating.
   d. increased alertness.

5. A major depressive episode is characterized by
   a. feelings of euphoria.
   b. rapid speech.
   c. profoundly depressed mood.
   d. inflated self-esteem.

6. A myth about suicide is that
   a. suicide attempts should be taken seriously.
   b. suicidal patients really want to die.
   c. suicidal patients are manipulative.
   d. suicidal patients are often depressed.

7. When a patient sees objects that are not there this is an example of
   a. delusion.
   b. regression.
   c. visual hallucination.
   d. tactile hallucination.

8. Signs and symptoms of amphetamine withdrawal are

   a. dysphoric mood; vivid, unpleasant dreams.
   b. euphoria, hyperalertness.
   c. anorexia, tachycardia.
   d. nausea, muscle aches.

9. Delirium has the following characteristics

   a. gradual onset, patient apathy.
   b. specific causes, memory impaired.
   c. acute onset, impaired attention.
   d. impaired memory, chronic condition.

10. An adolescent was admitted to the hospital with a weight loss of 15% of expected body weight. She has been refusing to eat. The most appropriate short-term goal is that the patient will

    a. divulge her concerns about her relationship with her family.
    b. gain 1-2 lb of weight per week.
    c. sign a contract not to purge.
    d. reduce her fear of obesity.

11. The primary reason a patient who is anorexic refuses to eat (but is preoccupied with thoughts of food) is that she

    a. is contemplating killing herself.
    b. suffers from pain when eating.
    c. identifies with thin models.
    d. is afraid of losing control over this aspect of her life.

12. The health care staff most at risk of work place violence are

    a. nurses.
    b. physicians.
    c. social workers.
    d. physical therapists.

13. When caring for a patient, if your _____ tells you that the patient may become dangerous, believe it, and seek help.

    a. anxiety
    b. intuition
    c. mental status
    d. fear

14. A legal concern with a noncompliant patient is whether the patient is

    a. acting mature.
    b. self-aware.
    c. knowledgeable about his rights.
    d. competent.

15. The primary goal of patient manipulation is to

    a. upset the staff.
    b. make the environment safe and secure.
    c. gain insight.
    d. gain empathy.

16. During the acute phase of cardiac illness, patients generally experience normal grief response. The most common response to myocardial infarction is

    a. denial.
    b. shock.
    c. anger.
    d. depression.

17. The following medications are used as a mood stabilizer

    a. lithium, carbamazepine (Tegretol®).
    b. carbamazepine (Tegretol®), phenelzine (Nardil®).
    c. zolpidem (Ambien®), diazepam (Valium®).
    d. lithium, amitriptyline (Elavil®).

18. Anxiolytics are used to treat

    a. depression.
    b. hallucination and delusions.
    c. anxiety.
    d. toxic reactions.

19. Veracity as an ethical principle means

    a. respect for the person to make individual choices.
    b. do no harm or minimize harm.
    c. truth telling.
    d. doing the greatest good for patients.

20. An example of a poor sleep hygiene practice is

    a. going to bed at the same time each day.
    b. commanding yourself to go to sleep.
    c. emptying your bladder before going to sleep.
    d. keeping the room quiet when sleeping.

INTRODUCTION

A basic premise of patient care is that patients who are being cared for by health professionals are undergoing some emotional stress. They may be anxious, have a serious illness, be in pain, or worse. Even the joyful occasion of giving birth is a highly stressful event that may be associated with some emotional sequelae. Patients with no previous psychiatric problems may experience emotional problems when they are hospitalized.

Some patients who have a psychiatric illness or a history of one may require hospitalization. A patient may need hospitalization because of an exacerbation of a psychiatric illness or its sequelae, such as sometimes occurs in people who are unsuccessful with a suicide attempt. In addition, psychiatric patients may experience illness or injury; they may break a leg, have a cardiac problem, or have cancer, to name a few situations. Nurses working in hospital or other institutional settings are in an ideal situation to help patients with emotional problems because they spend more time at the bedside than any other health care provider.

Patients who are undergoing emotional situations or crises require care that goes beyond the basic medical regimen. Nurses have a responsibility to deal with these problems in patients because it is part of their basic nursing care, however, this can present an increased challenge for nurses.

It is essential for nurses to maintain and update skills needed to care for patients who have emotional problems or are mentally ill in order to provide all patients with the best possible care. This course offers a guide to give you a broad overview of the care of patients who have psychiatric illnesses and emotional crises.

CHAPTER 1

THE COMMUNICATION PROCESS AND INTERPERSONAL SKILLS

CHAPTER OBJECTIVE

After completing this chapter, the reader will be able to recognize major components of the communication process and identify interpersonal skills that are used to ensure good nursing care.

LEARNING OBJECTIVES

After studying this chapter, the reader will be able to

1. explain the basic components of the communication process.
2. describe strategies and techniques that are used to facilitate effective communication.
3. discuss barriers to therapeutic communication.

COMMUNICATION

A basic premise of communication is that it is impossible not to communicate with one another. Nurse-patient interactions consist of both verbal and nonverbal communication. Effective communication can have a positive effect on nurse-patient relationships. It can increase patient's compliance with the plan of care and satisfaction level. It is important to develop communication skills that will work for you and your patients.

Process

Communication is an ongoing, dynamic and complex process. It is the transmission of feelings, attitudes, and behaviors from one person to another. People depend on verbal and nonverbal communication to understand their world and to communicate their needs.

Components

Three basic components are needed for communication to occur

1. Sender
2. Message
3. Receiver

Briefly stated, the sender delivers the message to the receiver. A simple example is the question nurses ask every day: "How are you feeling?"

1. The sender is the nurse.
2. The message is the question, "How are you feeling?"
3. The receiver is the patient.

The process is not linear; both senders and receivers simultaneously influence each other. Generally speaking, if a sender and a receiver are willing to communicate, a message will be conveyed and shared. The receiver's expression conveys a message of understanding, anger, or boredom when the sender sends a message.

Verbal communication involves an exchange of words, both spoken and written. Its basis is language, which is transmitted through speech received through the senses. It is an integral part of nurse-patient interactions.

Nonverbal communication takes on additional importance in health-related situations. Words do not convey the total meaning of what a patient or nurse is trying to express. Body language plays an important role in the communication process. What is said through gestures, facial expressions, posture, touch, eye contact, body movement, speech rate, and volume can be as important as spoken words. Mannerisms and even odors convey a message. Patients who arrive on a unit dirty, disheveled, and unkempt tell us without speaking that they cannot care for themselves at an optimal level. Sometimes patients ask questions that may be uncomfortable for nurses to answer. Sometimes nurses ask patients questions that the patients are unwilling to answer. When these situations occur, the nonverbal response in itself is a message.

For example, a woman whose terminal cancer has been diagnosed recently but who has not been told yet asks, "Nurse, am I dying?" The nurse, feeling unable to tell the patient the truth, does not respond at all. What do you think the patient feels? This nonverbal response may cause anxiety in the patient, because fear of the unknown is one of the greatest fears.

The nurse should make sure that the patient's communication has been understood correctly. Whenever possible, the message should be validated, because what is not being said may be just as important as what is said.

INTERPERSONAL SKILLS

Communication is at the core of nursing. Interpersonal skills are essential for every aspect of nursing. Nurses use communication skills to develop therapeutic relationships with their patients, families, informal caregivers, and health care providers. Obtaining information about your patients' thoughts, feelings, events, and views is essential to nursing practice. Simultaneously, your ability to establish a rapport with patients and being responsive to their needs will facilitate their ability to better understand their emotions and cope with their own reactions.

Communicating well and appropriately both to get a point across and to understand another person requires good interpersonal skills. All nurses can learn the skills of listening, understanding, and verbalizing. These skills allow nurses to respond more comfortably to the psychosocial as well as the physical needs of patients.

Therapeutic Tool

Psychiatric nursing skills are based on empathic listening, understanding the patient's internal frame of reference, and verbalizing emotional support and feedback, when appropriate. By applying these positive interpersonal skills in all their interactions with patients, nurses are serving as therapeutic tools. Just as cardiology nurses rely on electrocardiographic (ECG) machines for information, and surgical nurses apply sterile dressings to postoperative wounds to foster healing, psychiatric nurses use their interpersonal and communication skills to continually assess patients while simultaneously providing therapeutic intervention to care for patients' emotional and mental health. General hospital staff nurses are in a position to easily tune into the emotional status of their patients.

Considerations

Although the basic components needed for communication are simply a sender, a receiver, and a message, other factors also play a role in producing interactions that are accurate, successful, and positive.

Time. Communication is no better or worse during the day or the night, but the differences between these two should be considered. Illnesses, accidents, and mishaps occur at all hours of the day and night. Hospitals, nursing homes, residential treatment facilities, and some home health situations care for patients 24 hr a day. Most nurses work one of the three 8 hr shifts or one 12 hr shift per 24 hr in health care settings. At some point, every nurse probably has worked a night shift.

In most health care settings the pace that exists during the day shift when activity is plentiful, (such as patients being seen by consultants, physicians, and therapists; taken for tests; and visited by friends and family) changes dramatically during the night. Often patients are more anxious during the night, because they have fewer distractions (both people and activities) from their concerns and fears. This anxiety could be one cause of a patient's sleeplessness or of the increase in requests for nursing attention. When patients are awake at night, it is a helpful time for nurses to communicate with them.

Place. Where interactions occur also should be considered. Think about the environmental differences in the following health-related areas:

- Hospital unit
- Emergency department
- Operating room
- Nursing home
- Patient's private residence
- Physician's office
- Pediatric clinic
- Ambulance
- Psychiatric unit

These are just some of the health care settings where nurses interact with patients. It follows that different places may require different interpersonal skills for therapeutic interactions, because the needs of patients may vary.

Person. Although some of us have similarities, each of us is an individual. Each patient has unique feelings, thoughts, values, language, culture, attitudes, and personality. All of these factors must be considered when nurses and patients interact. Additionally, using the same words and phrases with all patients in all situations may not always be therapeutic.

Consider the following two situations:

1. A 35-year-old woman with severe abdominal pain is brought to the emergency department by her husband. She is crying and quite distraught. A nurse is able to take time to pat the woman's hand and say, "We're looking for what's wrong; we'll try to help you to feel better soon." The patient thanks the nurse for her concern.
2. A 35-year-old man drives himself to the emergency department. He says that he is having severe stomach pains, and his demeanor is stoic. During his workup, he is visibly grimacing, and he begins shouting for people to hurry up. A nurse approaches him and says, "We're looking for what's wrong; we'll try to help you to feel better soon." The patient yells at the nurse, "Do something and shut up." He pushes the nurse aside, says that all of the staff is incompetent, and clearly is beginning to lose control.

Although comforting words were of help to the first patient, the same words irritated the second patient. Consequently, nurses must assess each patient and situation individually and devise the appropriate communication strategy accordingly.

Situational variance. Patients who require health care may be anxious about their medical situation; different situations may require different interpersonal techniques. Patients in critical situations generally want and need swift and efficient care. For these patients, short communications delivered with a comforting demeanor are best.

Some patients may be out of touch with reality and misinterpret the words and actions of others. Interactions with these patients require special skills. A conscious awareness of choice of words is needed in these situations. When patients' needs are taken into consideration, therapeutic interaction and good communication are attainable.

STRATEGIES FOR EFFECTIVE COMMUNICATION

Effective communication is at the core of developing a therapeutic relationship with your patients. Certain therapeutic communication skills and strategies have proven to be more effective to demonstrate empathy and elicit the patient's perspective. Nurses should be aware of their demeanor and verbal abilities as well as their limitations. In situations of psychiatric and psychosocial stress, nurses need to use these interpersonal skills to accomplish a therapeutic outcome.

LISTENING

Listening and the therapeutic use of silence are valuable tools. Active listening is achieved by paying close attention to the patient's message. The nurse should attend to the patient's verbal and nonverbal communication. Facing the patient, maintaining an attentive posture, changing facial expressions to conform with the content of what the patient is saying, using hand gestures, and nodding and shaking one's head all convey giving attention. Some commonly used phrases that encourage interactions include:

- ah hah!
- uh oh!
- uh huh.

Silence is therapeutic when it is used to convey an interest in what the patient is saying. Sometimes nurses are uncomfortable with prolonged periods of silence. Listening without interrupting tells the patient that you want to hear more. It also allows patients to explore their feelings and thoughts, as well as for nurses to collect their own thoughts and formulate appropriate responses.

Feedback and Clarification

We have all had the experience of having spoken at length about something only to hear from the listener a question or statement that indicated that we were misinterpreted. Clarifying techniques help to make messages understandable. They help to reduce miscommunication and misunderstanding. Clarifying what is being said, heard, and understood by both parties should be an ongoing process in communication. Giving and receiving feedback helps to achieve this clarification.

Clear communication can be achieved by doing the following:

- asking questions
- answering questions
- summarizing what you have heard
- probing for more information, if needed
- giving more information as requested.

Reflection or paraphrasing can also be used to confirm what has been said. With this technique, the listener repeats in a questioning manner part of what has been said. Consider the following examples:

- You said that hurt?
- You could not hear?
- You're feeling nervous?

Reflection is a commonly used tool that successfully encourages patients to continue with what they were saying.

Questioning Techniques

Nurses continually need pertinent information from patients. Sometimes direct questions are appropriate. Consider the following examples:

- Are you in pain?
- Did you sleep last night?

In some situations, more often in the psychiatric realm, it is desirable to hear in detail what a patient is feeling and thinking. At these times, open-ended questions are helpful. Open-ended questions are phrased in such a way that they cannot be answered with a simple yes or no; they require some added content. Consider the following examples:

- And then?
- What do you mean by that?
- What happened next?
- Can you tell me more about it?
- When? Where? How?

Support and Reassurance

Care and nurturance are integral aspects of nursing. Providing support and realistic reassurance to patients at times of crisis is a valuable intervention.

Support and reassurance can be given through the use of comforting words, gestures, and facial expressions. Discriminating use of touch, such as a pat on the hand or a slight touch on the shoulder, and being at the patient's side are supportive measures. Essentially, you want to convey to patients that you understand them and are concerned for and interested in them, without offering false hope and promises.

Table 1-1 gives techniques that are therapeutic communication skills. Table 1-2 gives barriers to effective communication.

Learning therapeutic communication and interpersonal skills may take some practice. In all health care related situations, nurses should be aware of their demeanor and verbal abilities, as well as their limitations. They should use statements, phrases, questions, and gestures that are comfortable and natural for them. Particularly in situations of psychiatric and psychosocial stress, nurses need to use therapeutic interpersonal skills to accomplish a positive patient outcome.

TABLE 1-1: HELPFUL PHRASES FOR OPEN COMMUNICATION
Support and Reassurance
Good job! Nice work!
I understand.
You seem better to me today. How are you?
How frustrating for you.
What a difficult situation this is.
Feedback and Clarification
I don't understand.
I don't know what you mean by that.
I am not following your train of thought.
Did you mean _____?
What about that…?
I cannot answer that question, I am not comfortable answering you, or I'd rather not answer that.
Exploring, Questioning, Probing, and Interpreting
What are you feeling?
What are you thinking about?
You seem to be seeing things or hearing voices. Are you?
You seem angry.
It appears to me as though you have been _____.
Have you been thinking about hurting yourself?
Go on.
And then?
Tell me more about that!

TABLE 1-2: PHRASES THAT CLOSE COMMUNICATION

False Promises
I'll be back in a few minutes (not returning).

Rejecting and Disapproving
That's wrong.
Don't tell me that.
I don't believe you.
You can't be right.
It must be this way.

Challenging
You can't be seeing pink elephants.
There are no loud voices. You can't be hearing them.
If the FBI is after you, why haven't they caught you yet?
You don't look like God.

Defensiveness
How can you say that? Why, this is the finest hospital!

Discounting the Patient's Feelings
You can't be upset about that?
Everyone feels blue sometimes.

POTENTIAL BARRIERS TO COMMUNICATION

When nurses interact with patients, several problems in interaction and communication may arise that could create barriers to therapeutic effectiveness.

Foreign Language

In the United States, many people speak foreign languages, and some may never learn to speak English. Everyday, non-English-speaking people come to this country to live, work, or visit. Additionally, some states share borders with Mexico and Canada, where people speak Spanish or French as well as English. Some may understand English but not speak it well. Sometimes, elderly patients, someone highly stressed, in great pain, delirious, possibly demented, or psychotic may revert to their native language.

Generally, communicating with someone whose primary language is not English can make it difficult to obtain patient data and provide support. One error some nurses make is to speak louder to patients when they speak another language. This can be offensive, and does not help the patients understand English. Instead, speak slowly, and be careful to avoid jargon.

Possible alternatives include the following:

- Use an interpreter, preferably one with a medical background. Some institutions maintain a list of employees who speak foreign languages. Remember to address your questions to your patients, rather than the interpreter.
- If necessary, ask a relative or friend of the patient to interpret. In some situations, it is necessary to know the relationship between the patient and the interpreter, because the patient may be embarrassed, or unwilling to be truthful with the interpreter. Usually a family member is the best choice.
- Use facial expression and hand gestures as well as good body language when communicating.
- Use multilingual educational materials.

In a region that has many non-English-speaking patients, it is beneficial to learn their language or at least a wide range of the native vocabulary used in their care. A pocketsize translation book can be helpful. It is better to make an attempt to communicate with patients in their native language so they do not feel isolated, ignored, or anxious.

Ethnic and Cultural Issues

Patients with different ethnic backgrounds and other cultural influences require culturally sensitive care. Even though patients may speak English, their interpretation of language and the meanings ascribed to symbols, attitudes, and facial expressions, associated with different medical issues and procedures, may seem different from what is familiar to us. For example, patients from different backgrounds may respond to pain differently. Some are stoic; others need to "let out" their emotions.

Some cultures aspire to maintain dignity by not exerting independence. For others, the opposite is true, and maintaining distance from others is more the rule.

Some cultures use symbols, medicinal herbs and potions, and trinkets. Nurses need to guard against assumed similarity, denigration of differences, ethnocentrism, prejudice, and stereotyping. Understanding that a basic difference does exist, avoiding "jumping to conclusions" about the patient, and attempting to understand the cultural issues will help produce successful interactions.

Some persons have tremendous faith in their religion and request a visit from a member of their church. Others may have a belief in spiritual healing and cures and make use of ceremonial acts, rites, or visits.

You may want to try the following:

- Talk openly with patients. Ask them to explain what you might think of as "strange" behavior. Be nonjudgmental, observational, and curious.
- Ask others, such as visitors or coworkers, who may be of the same faith, culture, or background as the patient, about subjects that may confuse you.
- Become more knowledgeable about other cultures.
- Be open to others' points of view. It is not necessary to agree with them; just try to see things from their perspective and be empathic.
- When interacting, ask for feedback and clarification. Find out whether you understand correctly and whether you are being understood correctly. Ask the patient to repeat what you have said, and repeat what the patient says to you.
- Be flexible. Perhaps some health care facility routines can be changed or modified for the patient's benefit. This in turn helps the nurse.

Like people who speak a foreign language, patients of different cultural backgrounds may feel quite isolated in an unfamiliar environment. The nurse can be helpful by using interpersonal skills therapeutically.

Pain

Patients who are in mild, moderate, or severe pain may have difficulty maintaining interactions in a normal manner. The entire focus of attention of people in pain is generally upon themselves, their pain, and ways to seek relief. This preoccupation may create a barrier to the flow of communication. In this situation, nurses bear the burden of maintaining the interaction, of being flexible, and being able to forego interaction when necessary. They should be alert for cues that indicate the patient is willing and able to communicate and then communicate at those times.

Lethargy

Patients who are lethargic do not communicate as accurately and astutely as they normally might. Ways to overcome this barrier include the following:

- Assess the patient's level of consciousness.
- Ask the patient first if this is a good time to talk; then assess the patient's ability to maintain a conversation.
- Get feedback about the patient's understanding of what you are discussing.
- If the patient is too lethargic, wait for another time. The patient may be unable to sustain the interaction.

Mutism

Some patients pose a special problem because they do not verbally communicate, or they speak little and seldom. Some patients are mute and cannot speak because of a physical disorder or disability. Some psychiatric disturbances leave patients incapable of speech or unwilling to talk.

It is important to assess why a patient is not speaking. The reason may be included in the patient's records, known by the patient's friends or relatives, or conveyed by the patient in sign language. If a patient cannot speak, nonverbal gestures and written communications can be used. When a patient is unwilling to communicate, the nurse must consider why. Is the patient fearful and afraid; psychotic and not in touch with reality; desperately sad and depressed; or perhaps angry, hostile, and negative?

The following approaches may be useful:

- Make time to be with the patient. Try not to be rushed or too pushy.
- Set a time in advance to meet with the patient: "I'll be back in 15 minutes to sit with you. Perhaps you will share some of your concerns with me then?" This approach allows the patient to prepare for the interview. If you are not successful the first time, try again later.
- Sit quietly with the patient: "I'll just sit here with you and keep you company for a few minutes. We don't need to talk." This approach tells the patient you are willing to be with him or her without the pressure of speaking.
- Determine the appropriate amount of time to spend with the patient. Short, frequent contacts (for example, 5 min every 30-60 min) may be most comfortable for the patient and the nurse.
- Be supportive but not overbearing. Allow for some of the distancing needs the patient may have.

Interaction with a mute patient is obviously difficult. However, once the cause of the mutism is determined, you can plan for the best way to communicate with the patient.

Anxiety

Many patients experience anxiety on one level or another. Communicating with anxious patients requires some special attention. Patients who are highly anxious may not be able to pay enough attention to hear and interpret language correctly. Nurses are in a key position to help patients cope with their anxiety, which is reviewed in chapter 3.

Confusion

When patients are confused, it can cause barriers to therapeutic communication. Chapter 8 discusses the appropriate nursing interventions for patients who are confused.

Psychosis

Patients who are psychotic (i.e., out of touch with reality and perhaps delusional or hallucinating) cannot judge interactions appropriately. Chapter 6 provides more information on the nursing management of patients who are psychotic.

SUMMARY

Generally speaking, nurses who are empathic and who have a basic knowledge of therapeutic communication and interpersonal skills will communicate effectively with patients. Sometimes, nonpsychiatric nurses feel that they may say the wrong thing and thereby harm the patient or put words into the patient's mouth or thoughts into the patient's head. This is usually not the case. The techniques covered in this chapter are useful with all patients regardless of the patients' diagnosis and health care setting.

EXAM QUESTIONS

CHAPTER 1

Questions 1-6

1. The three basic components needed for communication are

   a. sender, listener, receiver.
   b. receiver, message, feedback.
   c. sender, message, receiver.
   d. feedback, listener, message.

2. The basic premise in communication is that

   a. the sender of a message is a nurse.
   b. we use body language.
   c. feedback occurs.
   d. it is impossible not to communicate with one another.

3. There are many techniques used in therapeutic communication. The phrase, "I don't know what you mean by that" is an example of

   a. feedback and clarification.
   b. rejection and disapproval.
   c. support and reassurance.
   d. exploring and defensiveness.

4. A psychiatric nurse's best therapeutic tool is

   a. sphygmomanometer.
   b. herself or himself.
   c. good assessment skills.
   d. good language skills.

5. A helpful phrase for open communication with a patient is

   a. "What a difficult situation this is."
   b. "No!"
   c. "That's wrong."
   d. "Everyone feels blue sometimes."

6. An example of a phrase that will close communication is

   a. "I understand."
   b. "Did you mean _________?"
   c. "Tell me more about that."
   d. "You can't be upset by that!"

CHAPTER 2

HOW TO ASSESS PSYCHOSOCIAL PROBLEMS

CHAPTER OBJECTIVE

After completing this chapter, the reader will be able to perform a psychosocial assessment and do a mental status examination on patients. The reader will also be acquainted with North American Nursing Diagnosis Association nursing and Diagnostic and Statistical Manual of Mental Disorders, Text Revision, diagnoses.

LEARNING OBJECTIVES

After studying this chapter, the reader will be able to

1. discuss the major components of the nursing process used as a standard in psychiatric nursing.
2. specify the components of a psychosocial assessment and mental status examination.
3. indicate nursing strategies for assessing psychosocial problems.
4. list NANDA nursing and *DSM-IV-TR* diagnoses.

THE NURSING PROCESS

Psychiatric nursing, although a specialty with its own standards of care as specified by the American Nurses' Association, uses a process consisting of systematic steps toward the delivery of care that are based on the science and art of nursing theory and practice. The process has four components:

1. *Assessment:* Gathering and analyzing verbal and nonverbal information through history taking and observation.
2. *Plan:* Establishing goals with the patient and developing strategies for achieving them.
3. *Implementation:* Using nursing interventions to attain goals.
4. *Evaluation:* Critically reviewing goal achievement: total, partial, or none.

The nursing process is an integral part of psychiatric nursing and of the delivery of psychosocial nursing care to all patients.

ASSESSMENT

Assessment of patients with psychiatric and psychosocial problems is a critical step in the nursing process. Sometimes nurses work with patients who are highly stressed, confused in thinking, or behaving in an uncontrolled, irrational manner. These situations call for interpersonal communications skills, and observation skills using one's senses, including hearing, smell, and touch.

- *Hearing:* What is the patient saying or not saying? Are there any strange noises?
- *Sense of smell:* Are any odors emanating from the patient or the patient's belongings or the room?

- *Sense of touch:* Touching patients is more common when they have physical problems which may require hands-on care such as dressing changes and physical rather than psychiatric monitoring. However, many patients have more than one problem.

Patient assessments are used to systematically collect biopsychosocial information to determine a patient's current and past health, functional status, coping skills, and to plan nursing interventions. All observations are valuable. The best strategy is to gather all the information available and prioritize it later when planning care. It is an ongoing process and does not exist in isolation from the other steps of the nursing process.

Each health care facility generally specifies which assessment tool it wants nurses to use. It is a standard procedure to thoroughly assess each patient when the patient first enters the health care facility. Although an entire assessment form need not be completed each shift, day, or week, observing changes in patients during each shift is part of the assessment process. If you did not admit the patient, it is also incumbent on you to review the admission intake summary provided by your colleague, and do follow-up assessments, as appropriate, of the patient's problems.

MENTAL STATUS EXAMINATION

The mental status examination (MSE) (Table 2-1) is as crucial to psychiatric nursing as the physical examination is to medical-surgical nursing. It is a comprehensive examination of a person's emotional state and thinking processes at a given point in time. The MSE is used by the interdisciplinary health care team as the foundation for assessing patients with mental health problems, and in making a diagnosis of a psychiatric illness. It focuses on the patient's current state in terms of thoughts, feelings, and behavior. The MSE helps to assess a patient's general appearance and behavior, speech, mood and affect, thought content and process, perception, orientation as to time, place and person, judgment, and insight.

Different formats are used. Some are quite detailed; others, such as mini-mental status examinations (MMSEs), are more abbreviated. Nurses who work in a facility that uses a standardized format need to become familiar with, and comfortable using, it. The information is incorporated in the nursing care plan and is part of a patient's medical record (Table 2-2 Example of a Mental Status Examination).

MINI-MENTAL STATUS EXAMINATION

An MMSE can range from finding out if the patient is oriented to time, place, person, and situation, to a more detailed format such as the Cognitive Capacity Screening Examination (Table 2-3).

A completed MMSE provides an extensive description of the patient's current emotional state and thought processes. In interpreting the data, however, it is important to consider the social and cultural background of the patient. Any given behavior may vary widely in its meaning, depending on the personal history and culture of the person.

PSYCHOSOCIAL ASSESSMENT

The MSE is only one part of a complete psychosocial assessment. The complete assessment includes a history-taking procedure and a nursing assessment that reviews the patient's past, present, and future goals, encompassing physical, psychological, and social components (Table 2-4). The psychosocial assessment is the foundation for

TABLE 2-1: COMPONENTS OF THE MENTAL STATUS EXAMINATION

General Appearance
Description of the patient's physical characteristics
Apparent age
Grooming
Hygiene (e.g., clean, dirty, disheveled)
Dress (e.g., neat, careless, bizarre)
Posture

Behavior and Psychomotor Status
Patient's body language, movements, and facial expressions
Stereotyped behavior
Gait
Gestures
Mannerisms
Movements: Types and speed (e.g., agitated, restless), tremors, coarse or fine psychomotor retardation, wringing of hands

Attitude Toward Interviewer
Patient's attitude (e.g., attentive, friendly or angry, dramatic or muted, cooperative, suspicious, hostile, passive, dependent, indifferent, seductive)

Affect and Mood
Description of the patient's emotional state
Affect: the patient's expression of his or her emotional state (e.g., facial expression)
Words used to describe affect include blunted, flat, normal range, constricted.
Mood: The pervasive and sustained emotion of the person
Words used to describe mood include sad, angry, happy, depressed, worried, nervous, suspicious, dull, hostile, elated, apathetic.

Speech
Characteristics of how the patient talks
Quantity
Rate of production
Quality
Words used to describe speech include pressured, rapid, talkative, lacking spontaneity.

Thought Content/Perceptual Disturbances
Assessments for disturbed thought processes or perceptual disturbances, or difficulty and strangeness in thinking, especially for two major problems: delusions and hallucinations.
Delusion: A fixed, false belief. For example, "The Mafia is out to get me", or "I am Jesus Christ."
Hallucination: False sensory data. Hallucinations can be visual, auditory, olfactory, gustatory, or tactile. The most common types are hearing voices or seeing visions or both.

Sensorium and Cognition
Orientation of the patient to time, place, and person: Essentially, we are asking if the patient knows who he or she is, where he or she is, and when this time is.
Alertness and level of consciousness: Does the patient's sensorium seem clear, or is it clouded and confused?
Memory: Assessment of three time frames
Immediate: Can be tested by asking the patient to remember three items for a few minutes; for example, "I am going to ask you to remember a key, a book, and a lamp; I'll ask you again later." Move on with other questions and then say, "This is a good time to try and remember the three objects I mentioned before."
Recent: Can the patient tell you, with considerable detail and accuracy, the events that led up to the hospitalization?
Remote: Refers to the patient's distant personal history. This type of memory is the most difficult to check for accuracy. Some simple questions may be ones about the patient's upbringing, where he or she lived, where he or she went to school.

General Fund of Knowledge
General information such as the name of the president of the United States, the name of the governor of the state where the patient lives, answers to simple mathematical calculations.

Insight and Judgment
Can be checked for by listening (1) to the patient describe what he or she thinks is happening to him or her at the present time and how he or she perceives his or her illness and (2) to what decisions the patient is making with regard to the current situation.

TABLE 2-2: EXAMPLE OF A MENTAL STATUS EXAMINATION

Interviewer: M. Nadler-Moodie, R.N. **Date:** ______________________

General Appearance: Elderly white woman, appearing her stated age of 69 years old, is dressed in a hospital gown, socks, and a bed jacket. Hair is gray and unkempt, she wears no makeup, her fingernails are long and dirty with some food particles.

Motor Status and Affect: When she is ambulating to the bathroom, the patient's gait is slow and unsteady. She is slightly tremulous and holds onto the wall for support. Her posture is stooped. Facies appear sad. She has poor eye contact, little or no smiling. Affect is blunted with low range, no spontaneity.

General Behavior: Patient lies quietly in bed, either sleeping or with her eyes closed. She's been wringing her hands.

Speech and Language: Speech is very soft and slow; she answers questions in monosyllables. No incoherence noted or any illogical or strange words elicited. Native language is English.

Mood: Often teary-eyed and appears to be depressed. When asked about her mood, she replies, "I'm just very tired, and I do feel a bit down."

Thought Content: Some difficulty concentrating. Denies any special thoughts, delusions, or hallucinations. Denies any suicidal ideation, but is morbid in her thinking, saying, "I'm old and sick, and I suppose I won't live very much longer."

Orientation: Oriented x 3: Correct on person and place, slightly off on date, thinking today is "9-24-89."

Memory: Recent memory fair to good. Can recall events leading to hospitalization. Remote: good recall of past history.

General Fund of Knowledge: Completed high school, gives information correctly, seems of average intelligence. Accurate on simple calculations; thinks abstractly to people in glass houses…responds, "You shouldn't criticize someone for doing something you do as well."

Insight: Insight seems poor: doesn't seem to understand the nature of depression as possible contribution to her declining health.

Additional Comments:

____

____

____

the nursing process, and although a great deal of information is included immediately, additional information can be obtained later on. Some patients may be too ill or confused to obtain a complete assessment at the time of your first contact.

Both the patient and the patient's immediate environment should be observed. Patients' belongings may tell us something about them. If a patient is alone, it provides us some social information. In all cases, we learn something about the patient.

In home care situations, a thorough assessment of the patient's environment is critical. Specific safety factors should be checked. Patients' general lifestyle and ability to care for themselves at home are ongoing considerations. An important consideration is their ability to manage their own medications. A great deal of information about a patient's

TABLE 2-3: COGNITIVE CAPACITY SCREENING EXAMINATION

Examiner ______________________
Date ______________________
Instructions: Check items answered correctly. Write incorrect or unusual answers in space provided. If necessary, urge patient once to complete task.
Introduction to patient: "I would like to ask you a few questions. Some you will find very easy and others may be very hard. Just do your best."

Addressograph Plate

1) What day of the week is this? ____
2) What month? ____
3) What day of month? ____
4) What year? ____
5) What place is this? ____
6) Repeat the numbers 8 7 2. ____
7) Say them backwards. ____
8) Repeat these numbers 6 8 7 1. ____
9) Listen to these numbers 6 9 4. Count 1 through 10 out loud, then repeat 6 9 4. (Help if needed. Then use numbers 5 7 3.) ____
10) Listen to these numbers 8 1 4 3. Count 1 through 10 out loud, then repeat 8 1 4 3. ____
11) Beginning with Sunday, say the days of the week backwards. ____
12) 9 + 3 is ____
13) Add 6 (to the previous answer or "to 12"). ____
14) Take away 5 ("from 18"). Repeat these words after me and remember them. I will ask for them later: HAT, CAR, TREE, TWENTY-SIX. ____
15) The opposite of fast is slow. The opposite of up is ____
16) The opposite of large is ____
17) The opposite of hard is ____
18) An orange and a banana are both fruits. Red and blue are both ____
19) A penny and a dime are both ____
20) What were those words I asked you to remember? (HAT). ____
21) (CAR) ____
22) (TREE) ____
23) (TWENTY-SIX) ____
24) Take away 7 from 100, then take away 7 from what is left and keep going: 100-7 is ____
25) Minus 7 ____
26) Minus 7 (write down answers; check correct subtraction of 7) ____
27) Minus 7 ____
28) Minus 7 ____
29) Minus 7 ____
30) Minus 7 ____

TOTAL CORRECT (maximum score =30) ____

Patient's occupation (previous if not employed) ______ Education ______ Age ______
Estimated intelligence (based on eduation, occupation, and history, not on test score):
Below average, Average, Above average ______
Patient was: Cooperative ___ Uncooperative ___ Depressed ___ Lethargic ___ Other ______
Medical Diagnosis: ______________________

IF PATIENT'S SCORE IS LESS THAN 20, THE EXISTENCE OF DIMINISHED COGNITIVE CAPACITY IS PRESENT. THEREFORE, AN ORGANIC MENTAL SYNDROME SHOULD BE SUSPECTED AND THE FOLLOWING INFORMATION OBTAINED.

Temp.	____	BUN	____
B.P.	____	Glu	____
Hct	____	Po_2	____
Na	____	Pco_2	____
K	____		
CI	____		
CO_2	____		
EEG	____		
ECG	____		

Endocrine dysfunction? ______________
T3, T4, Ca, P, etc.

History of previous psychiatric difficulty ______

Drugs: ______________
Steroids? L-Dopa? Amphetamines? Tranquilizers? Digitalis?

Focal neurological signs: ______________

DIAGNOSIS: ______________

Note: From *Screening for Organic Metal Syndrome in the Medically Ill.* by J. W. Jacobs, M. R. Bernhard, A. Delgado, & J. J. Strain. 1977, *Annals of Internal Medicine.* Reprinted with permission.

personal life, culture, likes, and dislikes can be observed from a home visit.

When assessment takes place in an outpatient setting, private office, or clinic, factors such as hygiene, grooming, and ability to travel to and from appointments are additional considerations.

NURSING STRATEGIES FOR ASSESSING PSYCHOSOCIAL PROBLEMS

Setting a Time Frame

It seems obvious that obtaining a thorough psychosocial assessment can be a lengthy process, and in nursing, time is precious. Therefore, a time frame should be chosen accordingly. Although an initial assessment done when the patient arrives is useful immediately, not all the information required needs to be obtained then. Some basic information can be obtained when the patient arrives, and the rest can be acquired later in a more relaxed manner. A rushed interview is doomed to failure, both in gathering information and in using the opportunity to begin establishing a rapport with the patient.

Ensuring Confidentiality

The most appropriate place for interviewing a patient is in private, so attempt to obtain the psychosocial history with as few people present as possible. If you are in a semiprivate room, close all curtains or dividers. Perhaps the patient is ambulatory or perhaps the patient's roommate might leave. There may be much information that a patient will be uncomfortable talking about in the presence of others, even family members or friends.

Patients deserve the right to confidentiality in what they tell you. You should reassure them about confidentiality at the beginning of the interview. You should advise them that the information would only be shared with the health care team. You should be careful not to divulge any information in

TABLE 2-4: COMPONENTS OF A PSYCHOSOCIAL ASSESSMENT

General Information
Includes demographic information and identifying data, such as
Name
Address
Date of birth
Sex
Race, ethnic background, cultural beliefs
Religion, background, beliefs, practices
Marital status

Presenting Problem
What is the patient's chief complaint? This generally is stated in the patient's own words, and should be quotable.

History of Problem
When did it begin?
What is the nature of the problem (e.g., signs and symptoms, concerns)?
Any events or occurrences that may have led to the problem?
Present therapeutic contacts (such as, therapy with physician, nurse, psychologist, social worker, other).
Has this problem occurred before?
Pertinent personal psychiatric history?
Pertinent family history?
Relevant past counseling?

Medical History
Past or present medical problems?
Pertinent family history?
Physician or other health-related visits?
Laboratory values: Any known, recent work on chart, other?

Socioeconomic Background
Family system
Occupation: Employment status
Education level: What was last completed school grade?
Financial situation: Include information on health insurance
Habits: Eating, drinking, smoking, drug use, personal hygiene

Sexual History
General activity
Preference

Support Systems
Friends
Family
Affiliations
Leisure time activity

Level of Stress During the Year Before Admission
Changes in work or school (e.g., promotion, demotion, firing, graduation, change of job or school)?
Change in the family (e.g., death, divorce, birth of new baby, child leaving home, change in residence, change in financial status)?

Normal Coping Ability
How does the patient normally cope?
What conscious coping strategies does the patient use when severely stressed?

Possible Questions:
"When you experience stress in your everyday life, what do you do to decrease it?"
"When you go through a very rough time, how do you normally handle it?"

Possible Normal Responses
Talk with someone.
Ignore it.
Withdraw.
Get angry and yell.
Get angry and be quiet.
Get angry and hit/throw something.
Drink.
Become anxious.
Become depressed.

Developmental History:
Include any pertinent childhood adolescent issues

Medications
Currently taking?
Past responses and reactions
Known allergies
Over-the-counter medications frequently taken

Significant Events
Any other occurrences, losses not yet mentioned?

an unethical manner. Patients should not be discussed with anyone who is not a participant in their treatment. In psychiatric settings, signed releases of information need to be obtained from the patient.

Documenting Findings

The nursing psychosocial assessment should be included in the patient's permanent record of care. This information will be read by other members of the multidisciplinary health care team.

Establishing Therapeutic Relationships

The initial intake period is the time to begin a therapeutic relationship with the patient, and establish trust. Show sensitivity and respect while communicating with patients. An empathic demeanor will indicate caring and interest.

An awareness of your own insecurities or anxieties about the patient should also be considered. Be alert to any potentially dangerous behaviors for the sake of the patient's safety as well as your own. If you are calm, patient, and interested, assessment can provide the foundation for therapeutic nursing care.

NURSING DIAGNOSES

As part of a complete psychosocial nursing assessment, nursing diagnoses have been used increasingly as one means of standardizing nursing practice. Nurses who are committed to achieving this standardization have established the North American Nursing Diagnosis Association (NANDA). NANDA publishes an updated list of nursing diagnoses on a biannual basis. The current list (2003-2004) has 167 entries (Table 2-5). The Association continues to research and develop new and refined nursing diagnoses as indicated by data collected.

DIAGNOSTIC AND STATISTICAL MANUAL OF MENTAL DISORDERS

The psychiatric diagnoses that are specified solely or along with medical diagnoses as part of a patient's permanent medical record are based on the *Diagnostic and Statistical Manual of Mental Disorders,* Fourth Edition, *Text Revision (DSM-IV-TR*; American Psychiatric Association, 2000). The diagnostic groupings most likely to be seen in general hospital nursing are as follows:

- Adjustment disorders
- Anxiety disorders
- Delirium, dementia, and other cognitive disorders
- Eating disorders
- Mental disorders due to a general medical condition
- Mood disorders
- Schizophrenia and other psychotic disorders
- Somatoform disorders
- Personality disorders
- Sleep disorders
- Substance-related disorders

CASE STUDY

The following case study describes a patient and presents the MSE as it might be written on a chart (Table 2-3). You are the day nurse on a medical unit. A woman was admitted to your unit last evening from the emergency department. Her diagnosis is pneumonia. She has begun taking antibiotics and has no complaints. You notice that she is crying, and she denies being in any pain. You feel that something is not right with this patient, and you make some time to do an MSE.

TABLE 2-5: NORTH AMERICAN NURSING DIAGNOSIS ASSOCIATION (NANDA) 2003-2004 LIST OF NURSING DIAGNOSES

- Activity intolerance
- Risk for activity intolerance
- Impaired adjustment
- Ineffective airway clearance
- Latex allergy response
- Risk for latex allergy response
- Anxiety
- Death anxiety
- Risk for aspiration
- Risk for impaired parent/infant/child Attachment
- Autonomic dysreflexia
- Risk for autonomic dysreflexia
- Disturbed body image
- Risk for imbalanced body temperature
- Bowel incontinence
- Effective breastfeeding
- Ineffective breastfeeding
- Interrupted breastfeeding
- Ineffective breathing pattern
- Decreased cardiac output
- Caregiver role strain
- Risk for caregiver role strain
- Impaired comfort
- Impaired verbal communication
- Readiness for enhanced communication
- Decisional conflict
- Parental role conflict
- Acute confusion
- Chronic confusion
- Constipation
- Perceived constipation
- Risk for constipation
- Ineffective coping
- Ineffective community coping
- Readiness for enhanced community coping
- Defensive coping
- Compromised family coping
- Disabled family coping
- Readiness for enhanced coping
- Readiness for enhanced family coping
- Ineffective denial
- Impaired dentition
- Risk for delayed development
- Diarrhea
- Risk for disuse syndrome
- Deficient diversional activity
- Disturbed energy field
- Impaired environmental interpretation syndrome
- Adult failure to thrive
- Risk for falls
- Dysfunctional family processes: alcoholism
- Interrupted family processes
- Readiness for enhanced family processes
- Fatigue
- Fear
- Readiness for enhanced fluid balance
- Deficient fluid volume
- Excess fluid volume
- Risk for deficient fluid volume
- Risk for imbalanced fluid volume
- Impaired gas exchange
- Grieving
- Anticipatory grieving
- Dysfunctional grieving
- Delayed growth and development
- Risk for disproportionate growth
- Ineffective health maintenance
- Health-seeking behaviors
- Impaired home maintenance
- Hopelessness
- Hyperthermia
- Hypothermia
- Disturbed personal identity
- Functional urinary incontinence
- Reflex urinary incontinence
- Stress urinary incontinence
- Total urinary incontinence
- Urge urinary incontinence
- Risk for urge urinary incontinence
- Disorganized infant behavior
- Risk for disorganized infant behavior
- Readiness for enhanced organized infant behavior
- Ineffective infant feeding pattern
- Risk for infection
- Risk for injury
- Risk for perioperative-positioning injury
- Decreased intracranial adaptive capacity
- Deficient knowledge
- Readiness for enhanced knowledge of (specify)
- Risk for loneliness
- Impaired memory
- Impaired bed mobility
- Impaired physical mobility
- Impaired wheelchair mobility
- Nausea
- Unilateral neglect
- Noncompliance
- Imbalanced nutrition: less than body requirements
- Imbalanced nutrition: more than body requirements
- Readiness for enhanced nutrition
- Risk for imbalanced nutrition: more than body requirements
- Impaired oral mucous membrane
- Acute pain
- Chronic pain
- Impaired parenting
- Readiness for enhanced parenting
- Risk for impaired parenting
- Risk for peripheral neurovascular dysfunction
- Risk for poisoning
- Post-trauma syndrome
- Risk for post-trauma syndrome
- Powerlessness
- Risk for powerlessness
- Ineffective protection
- Rape-trauma syndrome
- Rape-trauma syndrome: compound reaction
- Rape-trauma syndrome: silent reaction
- Relocation stress syndrome
- Risk for relocation stress syndrome
- Ineffective role performance
- Bathing/hygiene self-care deficit
- Dressing/grooming self-care deficit
- Feeding self-care deficit
- Toileting self-care deficit
- Readiness for enhanced self-concept
- Chronic low self-esteem
- Situational low self-esteem
- Risk for situational low self-esteem
- Self-mutilation
- Risk for self-mutilation
- Disturbed sensory perception
- Sexual dysfunction
- Ineffective sexuality patterns
- Impaired skin integrity
- Risk for impaired skin integrity
- Sleep deprivation
- Disturbed sleep pattern
- Readiness for enhanced sleep
- Impaired social interaction
- Social isolation
- Chronic sorrow
- Spiritual distress
- Risk for spiritual distress
- Readiness for enhanced spiritual well-being
- Risk for sudden infant death syndrome
- Risk for suffocation
- Risk for suicide
- Delayed surgical recovery
- Impaired swallowing
- Effective therapeutic regimen management
- Ineffective therapeutic regimen management
- Ineffective community therapeutic regimen management
- Ineffective family therapeutic regimen management
- Readiness for enhanced therapeutic regimen management
- Ineffective thermoregulation
- Disturbed thought processes
- Impaired tissue integrity
- Ineffective tissue perfusion
- Impaired transfer ability
- Risk for trauma
- Impaired urinary elimination
- Readiness for enhanced urinary elimination
- Urinary retention
- Impaired spontaneous ventilation
- Dysfunctional ventilatory weaning response
- Risk for other-directed violence
- Risk for self-directed violence
- Impaired walking
- Wandering

Note. From *Definitions and classifications, 2003 2004,* NANDA International, 2003. Philadelphia: The North American Nursing Diagnosis Association. Reprinted with permission.

While talking with the patient, you acquire additional information that is necessary for a more complete assessment. The patient says she has been sleeping a lot, has a small appetite, and cannot remember when she has been hungry for a full meal.

The chart reveals a history of early morning awakening; this is corroborated by the night nursing notes, which report that the patient awakened at 3:10 a.m. Her record states she has lost 5 lb (2.3 kg) in the past month.

The patient reports that she lives alone; her husband died 9 months ago. She has one son who lives 35 miles away and a daughter in another state. She speaks with them on the telephone but does not get to see them much. She has some friends but generally feels too tired to see them. She claims she is not a "joiner," and she does not participate in any community activities or church groups. She has always been a housewife, never working outside her home, and says, "I don't imagine I could do much of anything else."

Based on all of the data collected and the MSE, you accurately decide that this patient has a mood disorder, with signs and symptoms of depression. The nursing diagnoses include one or more of the following:

- *Impaired adjustment*
- *Ineffective coping*
- *Deficient diversional activity*
- *Imbalanced nutrition: less than body requirements*
- *Powerlessness*
- *Bathing/hygiene self-care deficit*
- *Chronic low self-esteem*
- *Disturbed sleep pattern*
- *Social isolation.*

EXAM QUESTIONS

CHAPTER 2

Questions 7-12

7. The four basic components of the nursing process are
   a. assessment, plan, implementation, evaluation.
   b. observation, plan, implementation, evaluation.
   c. communication, message, receiver, sender.
   d. plan, interventions, observation, assessment.

8. A patient assessment is important because it allows the nurse to
   a. report and document.
   b. provide support and reassurance.
   c. complete charting requirements.
   d. determine the patient's problem and plan interventions.

9. An example of a mini-mental status examination is
   a. asking if the patient is oriented to time.
   b. psychological history.
   c. Cognitive Capacity Screening Examination.
   d. DSM-IV-TR.

10. Components of a psychosocial assessment are
    a. medical history, treatment plan, confidentiality.
    b. language, orientation, sexual history.
    c. significant events, sexual history, motor status.
    d. general information, medical history, socioeconomic background.

11. An example of a nursing strategy for assessing a psychosocial problem is
    a. complete a nursing assessment.
    b. maintain good eye contact.
    c. establish a therapeutic relationship.
    d. perform a mental status examination.

12. A psychosocial NANDA nursing diagnosis is
    a. mood disorder.
    b. ineffective coping.
    c. anxiety disorder.
    d. obsessive-compulsive behavior.

CHAPTER 3

NURSING MANAGEMENT OF THE PATIENT WHO IS ANXIOUS

CHAPTER OBJECTIVE

After completing this chapter, the reader will be able to describe the concept of anxiety, and how it relates to caring for patients who are experiencing anxiety.

LEARNING OBJECTIVES

After studying this chapter, the reader will be able to

1. define anxiety, fear, stress, crisis, and posttraumatic stress disorder.
2. discuss the causes of and precipitating events and levels associated with anxiety.
3. describe the physiologic responses to, and, different levels of, anxiety.
4. list the NANDA nursing and *DSM-IV-TR* diagnoses pertinent to anxiety.
5. identify nursing interventions that may be effective with an anxious patient.

OVERVIEW

Most patients experience some anxiety about their health. Certainly, hospitalization is a stressor for anyone. Each patient experiences anxiety uniquely and behaves accordingly. When patients have difficulty coping with their current level of anxiety, you can help them reduce their anxiety by maximizing their coping abilities and/or using other stress reduction strategies.

DEFINITIONS

Anxiety is an unpleasant feeling of dread and apprehension. It may be caused by an unconscious conflict between an underlying drive and the reality of the environment, or it may be precipitated by a physical illness or a stressful situation. Patients who are anxious are often unaware of the specific cause of their feelings.

Fear is an unpleasant feeling caused by the realization and recognition that some event, occurrence, or other detectable source in the environment may bring harm.

Stress, classically described by Hans Selye (1976), is the natural occurrence of wear and tear on the body as it responds and adapts to life's events. Stress is generally recognized as a highly complex phenomenon. Accordingly, the definition of stress must emphasize the relationship between the person and environment, the situation and the person's physiologic state, the current event and the person's history of stress and coping, and so forth.

Both psychological and physical stress can precipitate feelings of anxiety. These feelings may be successfully coped with in a variety of ways, or they may be overwhelming. When they are overwhelming, the person's coping mechanisms may be insufficient to manage the anxiety.

Crisis is an internal disturbance that results from a stressful event or hazardous situation or a perceived threat to the self. During times of crisis, the patient's usual coping mechanisms become ineffective. At this point a patient is more receptive to therapeutic influence and can often learn new coping mechanisms. Fortunately, a crisis is a time-limited event.

CAUSES AND PRECIPITATING EVENTS

Some of the causes of anxiety and the precipitating events that lead to it may be unclear or unknown. It is generally related to situational or maturational factors or other factors related to the patient's basic needs for food, air, comfort, and security. Almost everyone experiences dread and fear of the unknown.

Everyone goes through maturational stages as part of normal growth and development and required role changes. These maturational states are developmental periods during which psychological disequilibrium can occur. Adolescence, marriage, parenthood, career changes, and retirement are examples of maturational crises.

Situational crises may be related to a specific external event that causes loss of a person's psychological equilibrium. Examples are a death of significant other, divorce, school problems, and illnesses.

The precipitating stressors are different for each person. Having an illness diagnosed as a dreaded disease or being injured can provoke an identity crisis. In addition to coping with the fear of the disease or injury itself, persons who are ill or injured may have to change their view of themselves.

Changes to a person's status are generally perceived as stressful. The event can be negative (e.g., an illness) or positive (e.g., the first day on a new job). The culmination of these events and feelings may become a crisis when a person's normal coping mechanism fail, and they no longer can cope effectively with day-to-day tasks.

Posttraumatic stress disorder (PTSD), an anxiety disorder, is the development of characteristic symptoms following exposure to an extreme traumatic event. It can result from a direct personal experience of an event that involves actual or threatened death or serious injury, or other threat to one's physical integrity, such as military combat, violent personal assault, or being taking hostage (APA, 2000).

PTSD can also result from witnessing an event that involves death, injury, or a threat to the physical integrity of another person, such as the plane hijackings and terrorist attacks on New York City's World Trade Center and the Pentagon in Washington, DC on September 11, 2001 (APA, 2000; Thobaben, 2002).

Additionally, PTSD can result from learning about unexpected or violent death, serious harm, or threat of death or injury experienced by a family member or other close associate (APA, 2000). The person persistently reexperiences the traumatic event, persistently avoids stimuli associated with the trauma, and experiences numbing of general responsiveness (APA, 2000). The person's response to the event involves intense fear, helplessness, or horror. The posttraumatic reaction can begin immediately, day, weeks, months, or even years after the traumatic incident (APA, 2000; Thobaben, 2002).

LEVELS OF ANXIETY

How anxiety effects a person's abilities will vary with the level of anxiety (Table 3-1).

TABLE 3-1: LEVELS OF ANXIETY

Level of Anxiety	Cognitive/Perception/Tension	Learning Ability
1. Mild	Alertness is increased Sensory input seems heightened Attentive Slight muscle tension	Logical problem-solving skills Able to achieve and succeed in specific tasks Can solve problem that is causing anxiety
2. Moderate	Narrowed perception Misperception of stimuli Ability to communicate is reduced Difficulty in concentrating Increased nervousness and tension occurs Moderate muscle tension occurs Increased pulse, blood pressure, and respirations	Some coping skills are still functional Can follow directions With some help, the anxiety can be dealt with successfully
3. Severe	Perceptual field becomes quite narrow Distorted perceptions Disoriented Focused on the short term Shortened attention span An accompanying physical discomfort may add to a sense of emotional discomfort Extreme muscle tension	Ineffective reasoning Ineffective problem solving skills Difficulty focusing on problem solving even with assistance Delusions with hallucinations if prolonged
4. Panic	Disorganized perceptions Has feelings of being overwhelmed, out of control, or terror Thoughts may be unfocused, random, fleeting, irrational, incoherent Severely impaired	Learning cannot occur Disorganized or irrational reasoning or problem solving Minimal functioning becomes difficult; Unable to reduce anxiety or solve the problem Cannot function at this level for long period

Four levels of anxiety are generally recognized. They range from mild anxiety to panic. When patients experience mild anxiety their perception and attention is heightened and they can learn. However, if patients' anxiety is at panic level, they cannot learn and are unable to function.

PHYSIOLOGIC RESPONSES

In addition to the many emotional changes that happen when a person is feeling anxious, several physical signs and symptoms may occur. They are generally experienced negatively:

- Abdominal distress
- Chest pain or discomfort
- Choking or smothering sensations
- Cold, icy hands
- Diaphoresis
- Dizziness
- Dry mouth
- Dyspnea

- Elevated blood pressure
- Faintness
- Frequent urination
- Headaches
- Increased respiratory rate
- Insomnia
- Nausea
- Palpitations
- Queasiness
- Restlessness
- Tachypnea
- Trembling
- Voice tremors

DSM-IV-TR DIAGNOSES

The psychiatric disorders generally associated with anxiety are as follows:

- Acute anxiety disorder
- Generalized anxiety disorder
- Obsessive-compulsive disorder
- Panic disorder with or without agoraphobia
- Posttraumatic stress disorder

NANDA NURSING DIAGNOSES

The NANDA nursing diagnoses for anxiety may include one or more of the following:

- Impaired Adjustment
- Anxiety
- Impaired verbal communication
- Decisional conflict
- Acute confusion
- Ineffective coping
- Defensive coping
- Fear
- Impaired memory
- Post-trauma syndrome
- Powerlessness
- Ineffective role performance
- Bathing/hygiene self-care deficit
- Situational low self-esteem
- Disturbed sensory perception
- Disturbed sleep pattern
- Impaired social interaction
- Social isolation
- Spiritual distress
- Disturbed thought processes

NURSING INTERVENTIONS

Patients can be helped to cope effectively during times of mild or moderate anxiety by having them use strategies that have been helpful in the past and other problem-solving methods of coping as needed. Patients who are experiencing severe anxiety or panic need help in coping and in reducing their level of anxiety to one at which problem-solving abilities can be effective.

The following nursing interventions may be appropriate for patients who are experiencing anxiety:

- **Intervention:** Establish trust, maintain a calm demeanor, and be nonthreatening.

  Rationale: To be effective with nursing interventions, establish a trusting relationship with the patient. Additionally, it is well known that anxiety is contagious. A patient's anxiety can affect the nurse and other staff members, and vice versa. Maintain a calm demeanor to be therapeutic.

- **Intervention:** Reassure patients of their safety and security. Staying with the patient, just being there, can provide comfort.

  Rationale: Patients may be experiencing a threat to their physical well-being or self-concept.

- **Intervention:** Communicate in a calm and clear manner with a succinct message and simple language particularly when the patient has a high level of anxiety.

  Rationale: When anxiety levels are high, patients may be unable to comprehend at their usual level of awareness.

- **Intervention:** Explore the patient's perception of harm and reality test the potential danger.

  Rationale: Clarifying the reality of the situation and assisting with the patient's coping mechanisms can reduce anxiety levels.

- **Intervention:** Decrease external stimuli by dimming lights, lowering background noise, and limiting the number and frequency of visitors.

  Rationale: External stimuli can increase anxiety levels.

- **Intervention:** Encourage verbalization.

  Rationale: By talking through some events and precipitating factors, patients can:

  - Gain insight into the precipitating factor.
  - Gain insight into their manner of coping with the anxiety itself.
  - Enact new strategies for coping.
  - Verbalize his problem.

- **Intervention:** Assist patients with skills they currently cannot master because of their anxiety.

  Rationale: When anxiety is especially high, usual tasks are more difficult, and learning new tasks is harder.

- **Intervention:** When the anxiety level has been reduced, explore the precipitating events.

  Rationale: A recurrence of anxiety may be aborted or reduced in severity when the patient can recognize the early signs and begin using strategies to reduce anxiety.

- **Intervention:** Teach patients to identify and describe feelings of anxiety.

  Rationale: When patients understand their experience of anxiety, they can:

  - Recognize the early signs and symptoms.
  - Perhaps reduce the level or thwart the episode.
  - Be receptive to adopting new coping responses.

- **Intervention:** Demonstrate and review available anxiety-reducing techniques, and help patients choose techniques and strategies to reduce their anxiety level. These include the following:

  - Relaxation techniques (e.g., breathing techniques, visualization, muscle tension reduction)
  - Physical exercise
  - Meditation and yoga
  - Occupational activity
  - Diversional activity

  Rationale: By reducing the level of anxiety, restoration of homeostasis is more obtainable.

- **Intervention:** Include the patient in setting goals and planning care.

  Rationale: Allowing patients a choice increases their chances of success and increases their independence and, therefore, their self-esteem.

- **Intervention:** Administer anxiolytic medications as prescribed, assess the need for medications to be given as needed (prn), assess the effectiveness of the drug, and monitor the patient for potential adverse side effects.

Rationale: Antianxiety medications can be beneficial in reducing the patient's anxiety for short-term use.

- **Intervention:** Teach the patient about the self-administration of anxiolytic medications.

  Rationale: The patient may benefit from anxiolytic medications and then continue taking them as an outpatient.

- **Intervention:** Assess the patient's mood, and observe for signs of depression and any possible suicidal ideation. If present, notify the patient's physician, and refer for ongoing psychiatric treatment.

  Rationale: Severe anxiety can coexist with depression.

CASE STUDY

Robert is a 22-year-old man who was admitted to an orthopedic unit of a general hospital with a fractured femur that has occurred while he was playing football. It is the first time he has had a serious injury. Robert recently had surgery to treat his injury, and his left leg is in a cast. He has an intravenous (IV) line and a urinary catheter in place. He is a big man and seems uncomfortable confined to the hospital bed. He has an order for Demerol (meperidine), 75 mg every 4-6 hr prn.

Twenty-four hours after surgery, Robert's nurse notices that he is restless. He calls for the nurse often because of minor complaints and seems to want a nurse in constant contact with him. His requests for pain medications exceed the order, and the night nurse reported that he slept poorly and complained often.

The nurse answers Robert's call-bell light and finds him crying and difficult to console. She approaches him, and he startles her by jumping upright in the bed, pulling at his IV line, and shouting some obscenities. Then he yells, "You just don't get it! This is driving me crazy!"

The nurse knows that Robert is having difficulty adjusting to both his injury and being in the hospital. She now approaches him more quietly. With a soft voice and with a calm demeanor, she asks him to describe what is bothering him. He tells her that

TABLE 3-2: PART OF A CARE PLAN FOR A PATIENT WITH ANXIETY

Problem No. 5

Date ______________________________

Problem/Nursing Diagnoses

Anxiety related to change in body image, as evidenced by tension, verbalized and demonstrated helplessness, verbalized fear, uncertainty, expressed concerns, grimacing, perspiration, sobbing, irrational behavior (e.g., pulling at IV, shouting).

Treatment Plan/Approaches

1. Assess level of anxiety.
2. Establish therapeutic relationship.
3. Offer appropriate interventions on the basis of level of anxiety.
   - **Mild:** Listen to patient, and redirect activities.
   - **Moderate:**
     Consider prn medications if ordered.
     Offer choice between two things.
     Try to decrease stimuli.
     Offer physical activity.
     Use matter-of-fact approach.
   - **Severe:** Stay with patient or check him often.
4. Help the patient recognize his feelings and describe what preceded them. If possible, connect the feeling to the unmet need; describe the patient's behavior, and connect it to the anxiety.

he is attending a local college. He gets good grades, and he hopes to graduate next June. He is co-captain of the football team and is considered a star player. After graduation, he plans to play football professionally. He is currently considering some offers. He begins to sob and tells her he is so upset that his ball-playing career has been suspended at this time and that he is worried sick over it.

The nurse correctly recognizes his psychosocial nursing diagnosis and adds problem 5, Anxiety related to change in body image, to his care plan (Table 3-2).

EXAM QUESTIONS

CHAPTER 3

Questions 13-18

13. An unpleasant feeling caused by the realization and recognition that some event, occurrence, or other detectable source in the environment may bring harm is

    a. fear.
    b. stress.
    c. crisis.
    d. anxiety.

14. Marriage is an example of

    a. stress.
    b. anxiety.
    c. a situational crises.
    d. a maturational crises.

15. This condition is associated with a person having a narrowed perception, moderate muscle tension, and the ability to follow directions

    a. mild anxiety.
    b. moderate anxiety.
    c. severe anxiety.
    d. panic.

16. Physiologic responses to anxiety include

    a. memory impairment, queasiness.
    b. choking, fatigue.
    c. restlessness, palpitations.
    d. chest pain, decreased pulse rate.

17. The NANDA nursing diagnoses of fear, ineffective coping, and decisional conflict are generally applicable for a patient who

    a. is depressed.
    b. is psychotic.
    c. has a personality disorder.
    d. is anxious.

18. The nurse explores the patient's perception of harm and reality tests the potential danger. These are examples of nursing interventions used with a patient that is

    a. critically ill.
    b. anorectic.
    c. depressed.
    d. anxious.

CHAPTER 4

NURSING MANAGEMENT OF THE PATIENT WITH MOOD DISORDERS

CHAPTER OBJECTIVE

After completing this chapter, the reader will be able to identify mood disorders and discuss how the principles of psychiatric nursing are used in the care of a patient with mood disorders.

LEARNING OBJECTIVES

After studying this chapter, the reader will be able to

1. indicate the prevalence of depression.
2. discuss the theories of causation and risk factors associated with mood disorders.
3. describe the treatments currently available for depression.
4. list the nursing and *DSM-IV-TR* diagnoses related to mood disorders.
5. identify NANDA nursing interventions commonly used with patients having mood disorders.

OVERVIEW

A mood disorder is an illness that involves the person's body, mood, and thoughts. It affects the way a person eats and sleeps, the way one feels about oneself, and the way one thinks. It is characterized by (a) extreme sadness, social withdrawal, guilt, and the expression of self-deprecating thoughts or (b) an elevated expansive mood with hyperactivity, pressured speech, decreased need for sleep, and impaired impulse control with poor judgment.

The former is called a major depressive disorder and the latter, bipolar disorder. When a patient's history indicates that both forms occur, the term used is bipolar I disorder. In bipolar II disorder, a patient experiences only hypomanic and depressive episodes, and not full manic or mixed episodes. During a hypomanic episode a patient experiences an abnormally and persistently elevated, expansive, or irritable mood that lasts at least 4 days (APA, 2000).

PREVALENCE

Depression is poorly recognized, and underdiagnosed. It is among the most treatable of psychiatric illnesses with estimates that between 80% and 90% of depressed patients respond positively to treatment. However, it first has to be recognized.

Sadness, hopelessness, nothing to live for, and despair — these words describe the feelings of depression. A major depressive disorder is an alteration in mood, a disturbance in a person's feelings marked chiefly by sadness, apathy, and loss of energy, making it almost impossible to carry on usual activities, sleep, eat, or enjoy life.

Depression is a serious biological illness affecting 9.9 million U.S. adults, or approximately 5% of the adult population in a given year (Cowdry,

2001). It is the leading cause of disability in the United States and many other developed countries. It can occur once in a lifetime or, for many people, it can recur several times. The most serious sequela of depression is suicide.

Bipolar disorder (also known as manic-depressive illness) is characterized by an alternating pattern of emotional highs (mania) and lows (depression), and can range from a mild condition to a severe condition. It affects more than 2 million American adults, or about 1% of the population age 18 and older. It often begins in adolescence or early adulthood and may persist for life (MFMER, 2002).

THEORIES OF CAUSATION

Different investigators have different opinions about the causative factors of depression. There is no doubt, based on the past decade of research, that depression and bipolar illness are brain disorders resulting from complex interactions among many biochemical, genetic, cognitive, behavioral, and environmental factors (NIMH, 2003). Some of the more widely known and accepted are the psychosocial and biological theories.

Psychosocial Theories

The psychodynamic or psychoanalytic view is that a loss or lack of love occurred when the person was a young child, and this experience has caused unresolved conflicting feelings and grieving. When these feelings go unresolved, the result may be feelings of rage, hostility, and anger turned inward. Thus, the person becomes depressed.

The cognitive theory, based on the work of Aaron Beck, author of *Cognitive Therapy and the Emotional Disorders* (1976), claims that depressive feelings result from faulty thinking, ideas, and beliefs; a distorted view of others; and a low self-esteem. When the person's thinking or cognition is corrected through cognitive therapy, the depression will be alleviated.

Interpersonal and environmental theories view depression as the result of a breakdown in communication with family and friends, problems with work, school, and carrying out general activities. Individual, group, and family therapies are used in this context.

Biological Theories

Research indicates that depression (as well as other psychiatric disorders) may be due to variations in levels of the biogenic amines. This theory relates to the catecholamines dopamine, norepinephrine, and serotonin and their functioning at receptor sites on brain cells and nerves.

Genetic factors also play a role in mood disorders. The prevalence of depression and bipolar mood disorders is higher among blood relatives than among the general population.

Ongoing scientific research is being conducted in the field of mental illness. Although no definitive cause has been found, more is known about the biological markers of depression now, and treatments are being used successfully.

RISK FACTORS

Illnesses

Some physical and mental illnesses and disorders have a cause-and-effect relationship with depression. Having a chronic illness, such as heart disease, stroke, or Alzheimer's disease, puts a patient at higher risk of developing depression.

The prevalence of depression is generally higher in persons who have concomitant medical problems such as the following:

- **Neurologic disorders**
  Neoplasms
  Stroke
  Multiple sclerosis
  Infections
  Trauma

Migraines

- **Endocrine disorders**
  Adrenal disorders
  Thyroid disorders
  Menses-related disorders
  Postpartum disorders
- **Infectious and inflammatory disorders**
  Chronic fatigue syndrome
  Pneumonia
  Acquired immune deficiency syndrome (AIDS)
  Tuberculosis
- **Other medical disorders**
  Vitamin deficiencies
  Anemia
  Cancer
  Cardiopulmonary disease
- **Nonmood psychiatric disorders that often coincide with a diagnosis of depression**
  Obsessive-compulsive disorder
  Panic disorder
  Substance-related disorders
  Personality disorders
  Eating disorders

Medications

Long-term use of certain medications may cause symptoms of depression in some people. Depression or mania is an idiosyncratic side effect of many medications, including the following:

- Hypertensive medication (e.g., reserpine)
- Sedatives, tranquilizers, barbiturates, and central nervous system (CNS) depressants
- Steroids (e.g., glucocorticoids, anabolic steroids)
- Cardiac medications
- Hormones (e.g., oral contraceptives)
- Amphetamines, including cocaine and crack, after the effects of these medications wear off

Stress

Stressful life events are difficult for some persons but may not pose problems for others. Loss or threatened loss of a loved one or a job can trigger depression. When assessing patients, the nurse should be aware of the patients' perceptions of their problems as a means of observing for signs and symptoms of depression.

Grief Reaction

Depression can be associated with loss and grief over a loss (e.g., anything a person valued, once had or wanted and now cannot have). This includes losing a spouse, parent, child, other family member, or friend to death or relocation. Situational grieving associated with events such as losing a job, divorce, and financial losses commonly are associated with a short-term depression.

Trauma

Some form of disaster or physical trauma, such as an accidental injury or a major illness, can precipitate an episode of depression.

Postpartum Depression

Up to 70% of women during the 10-day postpartum have "baby blues." It is transient and does not impair functioning. It should not been confused with postpartum depression, or postpartum-onset mood episodes (*DSM-IV-TR*, 2000).

Postpartum depression affects up to 25% of new mothers. It is caused by hormonal shifts, and/or inner psychological conflicts over becoming a mother for the first time, or once again.

Symptoms generally occur 3 days after the birth and usually within the first week and include sleep disturbances, increased anxiety, fatigue, irritability, or negative or ambivalent emotions toward and about the baby. The severity of signs and symptoms varies.

Less often, postpartum depression can result in a full-blown psychosis. The patient is profoundly depressed and suicidal, hallucinating or delusional, having homicidal thoughts or unreal feelings about the child (e.g., that the child is sick or dead).

Because of the brief time new mothers stay in most maternity units and birthing centers, nurses working on those units may not see the full extent of these disorders. Extreme or dangerous situations may result in the patient being readmitted, but usually to a psychiatric service. In the absence of life-threatening crises, attempts generally are made to care for patients at home. It is at home that the patient can have continuity in bonding and mothering her newborn, the comfort of a familiar environment and, it is hoped, family support.

New mothers may be irritable, anorectic, easily fatigued yet unable to sleep, and crying a lot. Fortunately, these episodes are usually self-limiting, lasting only a few days. However, the frequency of these signs and symptoms is high enough to warrant giving the new mother bedside education about them while she is in the maternity unit.

Nurses working in the community who may see new mothers in their homes a week or more after giving birth should be alert to the signs and symptoms of baby blues and its related psychiatric disorder.

Age

An increase in depression is noted in persons age 60 and older, and among older adults the prevalence of depression is generally 2 times higher in women than in men.

Some of the other high-risk factors for depression include the following:

- Physical illness
- A recent significant loss (e.g., the death of a family member or friend)
- An event such as a job loss and financial problems
- Unhappiness with one's occupation or having no job at all
- Low economic status
- Lack of social networks and social isolation

DSM-IV-TR CRITERIA FOR MAJOR DEPRESSIVE EPISODE

The signs and symptoms of major depression and the intensity of the feelings differ from person to person (Table 4-1).

The criteria for major depressive episode may include the following (have been present during the same 2-week period):

At least one of these two symptoms:

- Depressed mood
- Loss of interest or pleasure (*DSM-IV-TR*, 2000)

Additional criteria (need five or more):

- Depressed mood: feeling sad, empty, or irritable
- Loss of interest or ability to experience pleasure in usual activities
- Markedly diminished interest or pleasure in all, or almost all, activities
- Appetite disturbance: a decrease in appetite or overeating and perhaps even binging
- Sleep disturbance: insomnia, an inability to fall asleep or stay asleep, or hypersomnia, an excessive amount of sleeping
- Psychomotor agitation with an inability to sit still; continuous pacing and perhaps hand wringing as well
- Psychomotor retardation, feelings of fatigue, withdrawal, and low energy
- Low self-esteem, feeling worthless, exaggerated or inappropriate feelings of guilt
- Difficulty thinking or disturbed thought content, ranging from difficulty concentrating and making decisions to the extreme of delusions and hallucinations

TABLE 4-1: MOOD DISORDERS

Features	Major Depressive Disorder	Bipolar Disorder
Mood	Profoundly depressed mood	Feelings of euphoria; Extreme optimism; Liability of mood-altering between euphoria and irritability
Thinking	Difficulty thinking; Difficulty concentrating; Difficulty remembering	Distractibility; Flight of ideas; Thoughts are racing; Rapid speech; Inability to concentrate
Pleasure/Interest	Marked diminished interest in or pleasure from activities that were once enjoyed	Excessive involvement in pleasurable activities that have a high potential for painful consequences; Poor judgment; Recklessness
Weight	Significant weight loss or gain	Weight loss may be experienced
Sleep	Pronounced changes in sleep either insomnia or hypersomnia	Decreased need for sleep
Energy	Fatigue or loss of energy; Physical slowing or agitation	Excessive energy; Increase in physical activity; Psychomotor agitation
Self-esteem	Feelings of guilt; Worthlessness; Hopelessness; Emptiness	Inflated self-esteem
Suicide	Recurrent thoughts of death or suicide	Suicidal ideation may be present during a depressive episode

Note. From *Mood Disorders. Diagnostic and Statistical Manual of Mental Disorders,* Fourth Edition, Text Revision, by the American Psychiatric Association. 2000, Washington, DC: American Psychiatric Association. Reprinted with permission.

- Recurrent thoughts of death or suicidal ideations, plans, or attempts
- Diminished or no sexual desire (DSM-IV-TR, 2000)

It is important for nonpsychiatric nurses to be aware of the significance of depression among general hospital patients. They may complain of a variety of physical complaints, such as gastrointestinal problems (indigestion, constipation, and diarrhea), headache, and backache. Additionally, persistent physical symptoms that do not respond to treatment, such as headaches, gastrointestinal disorders, and chronic pain may indicate depression.

DSM-IV-TR CRITERIA FOR MANIC EPISODE

Bipolar I disorder is a mood disorder in which the person experiences episodes of mania or hypomania (less intense form of mania). The severity of signs and symptoms in each episode varies from person to person (Table 4-1).

The criteria for manic episode may include the following (lasting at least 1 week):

Must have:

Abnormally and persistently elevated, expansive or irritable mood (*DSM-IV-TR*, 2000).

Additional criteria (need three or more):

- Inflated self-esteem, grandiosity
- Decreased need for sleep, physical restlessness
- More talkative than usual; rapid, pressured speech; flight of ideas with racing thoughts

- Distractibility
- Easily disturbed
- Increased goal-oriented activity or psychomotor agitation
- Excessive involvement in pleasurable activities that have a high potential for painful consequences, such as hypersexuality (*DSM-IV-TR*, 2000)

TREATMENT OPTIONS

Different types of treatments are used for patients with depression, and consideration is given to the patient's history and severity of signs and symptoms. In general, a combination of some form of psychotherapy and an antidepressant medication is the preferred treatment.

Psychotherapies

Psychotherapy, a goal-oriented approach aimed at helping patients deal with a specific issue, is used in both inpatient and outpatient settings on short- and long-term bases. Patients may be treated individually, within groups, or with family members.

Scientific evidence indicates that several forms of short-term psychotherapy (cognitive, interpersonal, and behavioral) are effective in treating most cases of mild or moderate depression.

Treatments are based on a variety of theories, such as systems theory, communications theory, and interpersonal theory.

Long-term psychotherapy is seldom necessary to treat depression because psychopharmacologic therapy is so effective.

Somatic Treatments

Psychopharmacologic therapy

Depression: With estimated efficacy rates of 70-80%, psychopharmacologic therapy is a popular form of treatment of depression. Since the 1960s, the use of tricyclic antidepressants and monoamine oxidase inhibitors in combination with psychotherapy has constituted the principal mode of treatment.

Presently selective serotonin reuptake inhibitors such as fluoxetine (Prozac®, Sarafem®), paroxetine (Paxil®), sertraline (Zoloft®), and citalopram (Celexa®) are the first-line treatment for depression because they work faster and have fewer serious side effects than the older drugs.

Generally, tricyclic antidepressants take 2-3 weeks to produce therapeutic results. They are sometimes prescribed to treat moderate to severe depression. They include amitriptyline (Elavil®, Endep®), desipramine (Norpramin®, Pertofrane®), nortriptyline (Aventyl®, Pamelor®), protriptyline (Vivactil®), trimipramine (Surmontil®) and a combination of perphenazine and amitriptyline (Triavil®, Etrafon®). Tetracyclines include maprotiline (Ludiomil®) and mirtazapine (Remeron®).

The monoamine oxidase inhibitors, phenelzine (Nardil®) and tranylcypromine (Parnate®), prevent the breakdown of neurotransmitters. They are usually only used when other options have failed, because they have potentially serious side effects if combined with certain other medications or food products.

Often the patient is improved after the first few weeks of taking antidepressant medications; however, it must be taken regularly for 3-4 weeks (sometimes as many as 8 weeks) before the full therapeutic effect occurs (MFMER, 2003).

Bipolar disorder: Persons who have bipolar disorder are generally treated with lithium (Eskalith®, Lithobid®), valproic acid (Depakene®), divalproex (Depakote®), and carbamazepine (Epitol®, Tegretol®, Carbatrol®). It is effective in the management and stabilization of the illness in 50-80% of the time (MFMER, 2003). Patients who are taking lithium carbonate must have their serum levels of the drug monitored closely. The medication must be taken continuously; its effectiveness is contingent on maintaining a therapeutic blood level.

Electroconvulsive therapy

Electroconvulsive therapy (ECT) can be an effective treatment for the alleviation of depression. Generally, it is used only after a trial of antidepressants has failed or for patients at high risk for suicide.

During the procedure the patient is anesthetized and a seizure is induced. Treatments are given in a series of 6-10 over 2-3 weeks. ECT is primarily indicated for major depressive disorder.

Although the short-term memory loss associated with this type of therapy is well known, more profound and longer lasting adverse effects are rare. It is usually used for people who don't respond to medications, for those at high risk of suicide, and for severely depressed older adults who can't take medications because of heart disease (MFMER, 2003).

In some health care settings, nurses may assist with the administration of ECT on an inpatient or outpatient basis and provide nursing care to the patient who has received ECT.

On a home visit, an outpatient clinic or office visit, the nurse would need to monitor the effects and side effects of treatment for patients who have had ECT.

DSM-IV-TR DIAGNOSES

The *DSM-IV-TR* diagnostic categories for depression are listed under the umbrella category of mood disorders. The nurse may find one of the following psychiatric diagnoses among the patient's medical diagnoses in the patient's record:

- Depressive disorders
  - Major depressive disorder
  - Dysthymic disorder
- Bipolar disorders
  - Bipolar I disorder
  - Bipolar II disorder
  - Cyclothymic disorder

NANDA NURSING DIAGNOSES FOR MAJOR DEPRESSIVE AND BIPOLAR DISORDERS

NANDA nursing diagnoses for mood disorders may include one or more of the following:

- Anxiety
- Impaired verbal communication
- Ineffective coping
- Anticipatory grieving
- Dysfunctional grieving
- Hopelessness
- Risk for injury
- Unilateral neglect
- Noncompliance
- Imbalanced nutrition: less than body requirements
- Imbalanced nutrition: more than body requirements
- Post-trauma syndrome
- Risk for post-trauma syndrome
- Powerlessness
- Ineffective role performance
- Bathing/hygiene self-care deficit
- Dressing/grooming self-care deficit
- Feeding self-care deficit
- Toileting self-care deficit
- Chronic low self-esteem
- Situational low self-esteem
- Risk for situational low self-esteem

- Disturbed sensory perception
- Sleep deprivation
- Disturbed sleep pattern
- Impaired social interaction
- Social isolation
- Disturbed thought processes
- Risk for other-directed violence
- Risk for self-directed violence

NURSING INTERVENTIONS

Patients in a general hospital setting may experience a mood disorder. They may be receiving treatment for the disorder before or during their hospital stay.

Nursing interventions for patients who have mood disorders are quite effective in helping the patients maintain a psychosocial balance while in the hospital and perhaps in helping them take steps for ongoing care. Nurses who administer care at the bedside can provide valuable assistance to these patients by using some of the following nursing interventions.

- **Intervention:** Be accepting. The patient may have a negative outlook and low self-esteem.

  Rationale: An attitude of acceptance enhances feelings of self-worth.

- **Intervention:** Be nonjudgmental, develop a trusting relationship, and be open with the patient.

  Rationale: Trust is basic to a therapeutic relationship.

- **Intervention:** Assess the patient often.

  Rationale: Depressed patients need short frequent contacts to assure them that they are supported, safe, and attended to, even when they may feel that they are not worth your attention.

- **Intervention:** Screen patients for depression by asking:

  - During the past 2 weeks, have you felt down, depressed, or hopeless?
  - During the past 2 weeks, have you felt little interest or pleasure in doing things? (AHRQ, 2002; Thobaben, 2002)

  Rationale: The U.S. Preventive Services Task (*Agency for Healthcare Research and Quality* [AHRQ]) found that asking the previous two questions was an effective screening method to screen for depression. If your patient responds positively to the two questions, you can inform their physician, and they can receive appropriate treatment for depression.

- **Intervention:** Assess the patient for suicidal ideation, and initiate safety checks and procedures as needed.

  Rationale: Patients with depression may have suicidal feelings and thoughts. They may need protection from harm.

- **Intervention:** Assess the patient for any indications of a thought disorder.

  Rationale: Some patients with depression have accompanying psychotic thoughts.

- **Intervention:** Assess the patient's ability to perform self-care tasks.

  Rationale: Depression may decrease a person's ability to continue usual activities of daily living.

- **Intervention:** Assess the patient's sleep patterns and determine methods to either reduce or increase sleep, for example, using relaxation techniques, decreasing stimulation at rest time, and drinking warm milk.

  Rationale: Disturbances in sleep patterns are common in patients with depression or bipolar disorder.

- **Intervention:** Reduce the environmental stimuli for patients experiencing a hypomanic or manic episode.

Rationale: Patients are generally quite easily distracted when they are manic.

- **Intervention:** Provide structure and set limits as guides for a manic patient.

  Rationale: Generally, manic patients show poor judgment and impulsivity; they may need guidance.

- **Intervention:** Provide the patient an opportunity to express pent-up emotions or discuss problems (e.g., grieving a loss, internal mood, isolation, dysfunctional thinking).

  Rationale: If patients recognize possible precipitating events, they can take steps to:

  - Reduce occurrence of the events.
  - Devise strategies that may reduce or eliminate the stressors.

- **Intervention:** Allow the patient to cry in a supportive environment.

  Rationale: The patient may relieve pent-up feelings by crying.

- **Intervention:** Help the patient determine appropriate ways of expressing anger.

  Rationale: Patients with a moderate amount of depression are often angry.

- **Intervention:** Assist the patient in problem solving.

  Rationale: Problem solving reduces stresses and increases the patient's self-esteem.

- **Intervention:** Encourage patients to make their own choices when they experience feelings of powerlessness.

  Rationale: Patients gain a sense of control and mastery when they make choices.

- **Intervention:** Encourage patients to increase their interpersonal contacts.

  Rationale: Interpersonal relationships can reduce feelings of social isolation.

- **Intervention:** Administer prescribed medications.

  - Assess the effectiveness of the medication.
  - Monitor the patient for potential side effects.

  Rationale: Medications are an effective treatment for depression or bipolar disorder.

- **Intervention:** Teach the patient about the self-administration of prescribed medications.

  Rationale: Although quite beneficial for many patients, medications are quite potent and must be monitored carefully.

- **Intervention:** If the patient has experienced a loss, describe the stages of grieving and teach the patient about them.

  Rationale: Knowledge of the process of normal grieving helps patients accept their own feelings.

CASE STUDY

Mrs. Lenox is a 47-year-old woman who was admitted to a surgical unit of a general hospital for removal of an ovarian cyst. The procedure went well and medically Mrs. Lenox is doing fine.

The evening nurse was with the patient and noted that she seemed depressed. The patient and her husband divorced last year. Her second child, a daughter, left for college in the past 2 months, and her oldest child, a son, is married and living 500 miles away. Mrs. Lenox admitted that she has been feeling sad, having frequent crying spells, having a poor appetite, and being more tired than usual. She claims that she falls asleep easily at about 11 p.m. each night but finds herself wide awake at 2 a.m., unable to return to sleep and feeling quite dreadful.

The nurse accurately diagnoses the problem as depression and over the course of the next few days does the following:

- *Discusses her findings with Mrs. Lenox's physician, who agrees.*
- *Assesses for changes in behavior indicative of depression: saddened face, crying spells, feel-*

ings of dread, poor appetite, and early morning awakening.

- *Makes additional time to spend with Mrs. Lenox, encouraging verbalization.*
- *Teaches Mrs. Lenox the signs and symptoms of depression.*
- *Makes a referral for professional psychiatric assessment.*

SUMMARY

Because nurses spend so much time with patients, they are in a strategically important place for assessing a patient's mood. Patients who have a mood disorder are seen regularly in the general hospital. Nurses can take appropriate steps to ensure that patients receive appropriate treatment while in the hospital and after discharge.

EXAM QUESTIONS

CHAPTER 4

Questions 19-24

19. Depression is a serious biological illness affecting approximately what percent of the adult population in a given year?

    a. 25.

    b. 10.

    c. 5.

    d. 1.

20. Interpersonal theorists view depression as

    a. an incomplete cognition.

    b. a biochemical imbalance.

    c. the result of an event in childhood.

    d. a breakdown in communication with family and friends.

21. Bipolar disorder is

    a. a mood disorder with bouts of highs and lows.

    b. a life-threatening illness.

    c. baby blues.

    d. a major depression.

22. The treatment of choice for a patient with severe persistent depression who is dangerously suicidal is

    a. long-term analytic treatment.

    b. electroconvulsive therapy.

    c. crisis intervention.

    d. antipsychotic medications.

23. A nursing diagnosis for patient with depression is

    a. alteration in mood.

    b. mood disorder.

    c. risk for self-directed violence.

    d. alteration in affect.

24. Administering prescribed medications is an example of a (an)

    a. nursing intervention.

    b. medical intervention.

    c. crisis intervention.

    d. alteration in mood.

CHAPTER 5

NURSING MANAGEMENT OF THE SUICIDAL PATIENT

CHAPTER OBJECTIVE

After completing this chapter, the reader will be able to assess a patient for suicidal ideation and specify nursing interventions that may be beneficial in caring for such a patient.

LEARNING OBJECTIVES

After studying this chapter, the reader will be able to

1. indicate the prevalence of suicide in the United States.
2. discuss the risk factors for predicting which patients may be suicidal.
3. recognize myths that nurses may have about persons who attempt suicide.
4. list the NANDA nursing and *DSM-IV-TR* diagnoses related to the suicidal patient.
5. identify nursing interventions commonly used with patients who have suicidal ideation.

OVERVIEW OF THE PROBLEM

Suicide is the most common serious sequela of the mental and emotional disorders. It is the final and most drastic step toward attempting to cope, manage, or deal with one or more perceived threats to the self, whether they are biological, psychological, or emotional.

Nurses in the general hospital may care for patients who are suicidal for a variety of reasons. Patients who are unsuccessful in their suicide attempt may be hospitalized because of a shooting, cutting, carbon monoxide poisoning, or an overdose. Those who survive a suicide attempt often are brought to a general hospital emergency department, where they receive medical treatment before or at the same time as their psychiatric treatment. Additionally, severely depressed patients may attempt suicide while hospitalized. Nurses who work in outpatient settings, clinics, offices, or home care may assess that a patient is suicidal or confront the outcome of a failed attempt.

PREVALENCE

Accurate data and statistics on the rate of suicide are difficult to gather because suicide continues to be veiled by stigma. Some suicides are not reported, and some causes of death are recorded inaccurately.

The Centers for Disease Control and Prevention (CDC, 2003) reports that more than 29,000 people in the United States die by suicide every year. It is this country's 11th leading cause of death. It accounts for 1.3% of all deaths.

A person dies by suicide about every 18 minutes and an attempt is estimated to be once a minute. Every day, approximately 86 people take their own life, and 1,500 attempt. Eight to 25 attempted suicides are made to one completion (CDC, 2003).

THEORIES OF CAUSATION

Suicide is not a new phenomenon. Diverse and complex factors contribute to any particular suicide. The suicidal person may be any age, male or female, rich or poor. No culture is immune, and no race or religion is protected. There is, however, a lack of consensus as why do people want to die. Several theories of causation have been formulated.

Psychodynamic theorists believe that suicide is anger and aggression turned inward. It is a sadomasochistic act; people who commit suicide punish themselves and those who love them. A related idea is that the only way suicidal persons can gain some control over themselves or their particular situation is to kill themselves, thereby showing some mastery over their own fate.

Two other theoretical models of suicide are The Overlap Model and The Three Element Model. The Overlap Model predicts that the greater the area of overlap of risk factors from varying domains (biology, heredity, and life events), the more likely a person is to commit suicide. The Three Element Model emphasizes the combination of predisposing factors, family history, social environment, personality, life situation, and availability of suicide mechanisms, such as firearms (Laux 2002).

RISK FACTORS

Demographics

Age, sex, and race should be considered. Statistics show that elderly people and whites are more likely than younger people or nonwhites to commit suicide, and more men than women succeed at suicide, although more women attempt it. According to the CDC

- There are more than four male suicides for every one female suicide.
- Twice as many females as males attempt suicide.
- White men age 85 and older have a suicide rate that is 6 times that of the overall national rate.
- The suicide rates for women peak between ages 45-64, and do so again after age 75.
- For persons between ages 15-24, it is the third leading cause of death, behind unintentional injury and homicide (CDC, 2003).

Most elderly patients who complete suicide see their physicians within a few months of their death and more than one-third within the week of their suicide. Risk factors for suicide among elderly people include

- the presence of a mental illness — especially depression and alcohol abuse
- the presence of a physical illness
- social isolation — especially being widowed in males
- the availability of firearms in the home (AFFSP, 2003).

Personal History

Collecting data related to self-descriptive behavior is essential. Has the person attempted suicide in the past? If so, how many times, how often, and how lethal was the method? People who have previously attempted suicide and are again in crisis are more likely to attempt suicide again. Has a family member committed suicide? Having a history of a family member or close friend commit suicide increases a person's risk for self-inflicted death.

Social Factors

The prevalence of suicide is high among persons who are socially isolated, withdrawn, or independent, and among persons with little or no religious affiliation. Some religions hold strict beliefs against suicide. They consider suicide a sin, and this belief may make a difference in whether or not a person considers it as an option. Suicide also occurs more often among the unemployed, those forced to retire, young people from broken homes, and those whose families are in discord.

Resources

Does the patient have any family, friends, community organizations, or groups of any sort with which he is attached to or affiliated? Is the patient in communication with others on a regular basis? These factors may be helpful in discouraging suicidal thoughts.

Psychiatric and Medical Illness Factors

Persons with thoughts of harming themselves are overwhelmed by unbearable emotions. Patients who are suicidal often feel as though life is no longer worth living because they find no meaning in their own existence. They may have distorted thinking, be psychotic, confused, or under the influence of drugs or alcohol. Although there is no definite way to predict who may attempt suicide, a number of precipitating factors are associated with many suicides and therefore are considered high-risk factors.

Suicide is a potential solution for patients who are severely depressed. They can experience the following emotions:

- despair
- guilt
- shame
- hopelessness
- helplessness
- extreme weariness.

Patients who have serious medical problems with severe pain or a terminal illness may see no other way out for themselves and may think of suicide as a release. Some patients with multiple problems have few or no coping skills and cannot see any solutions to the problems. Others may feel an overwhelming sense of responsibility for someone else's unhappiness (e.g., a spouse, parent, or child) and think this other person would be better off without them. Whatever the person's situation, the emotions are generally deep and overwhelming.

The vast majority of patients who have attempted or completed suicide have an associated major psychiatric illness: mood disorders, substance-related disorders, and schizophrenia are the most frequently seen.

The following statistics are particularly noteworthy:

- Over 60% of all people who die by suicide suffer from major depression.
- Alcoholism is a factor in about 30% of all completed suicides.
- In alcoholics who are depressed, this figure rises to over 75%.
- People with AIDS have a suicide risk up to 20 times that of the general population (AFFSP, 2003).

MYTHS

Although it is almost impossible to predict who will commit suicide, some widespread myths do exist (Table 5-1). A common myth is that people who talk about suicide will never actually kill themselves. This belief is generally the opposite of what really happens. Most people who attempt suicide do talk about their suicidal feelings or give clues about their despondency. According to estimates, this group includes approximately 80% of successful suicides. Most suicidal persons have some ambivalence and feel a need to express feelings of despair and confusion.

Some medical personnel believe that a suicide threat is just a means to get some attention.

TABLE 5-1: COMMON MYTHS ABOUT SUICIDE
People who talk about suicide rarely commit it All threats must be taken seriously, the patient usually gives some clue or warning about their despondency.
Suicide is inherited A family history of suicide does increase one's risk, but there is no suicide gene that is inherited.
Suicidal people really want to die Patients are actually ambivalent about death, and frequently call for help after a suicide attempt.
Asking someone directly about suicidal ideation will encourage them to make a suicide attempt Talking with patients will encourage them to verbalize their concerns rather than acting them out, and will help decrease their social isolation.

Although it is true that a suicide attempt is a cry for help, each person's mind is complex, and all suicidal threats should be taken seriously. Some nurses think that they will plant suicidal ideas into the brain of a distraught person by merely mentioning or asking about suicide during an interaction or assessment. This belief is false. If a nurse thinks a patient may be suicidal, assessment of the patient must include direct questions about suicide.

ASSESSMENT

Although no absolute predictive measures are available, a careful assessment can provide enough information to protect the patient immediately and long term assistance can then be sought. Patients who are thought to be suicidal need careful monitoring and assessment of their suicidal potential.

- If a nurse thinks a patient may be suicidal, the nurse should ask. This can be phrased in many ways:
  - Are you thinking of killing yourself?
  - Do you just want to end it all?
  - Have you been considering ways to harm yourself?
  - Do you feel like hurting yourself?
  - Do you mean you are feeling suicidal?
  - Have you been thinking of hurting yourself?
- Sometimes patients leave guarded or veiled messages, perhaps a note or a letter. Suicidal patients may suddenly give away valuable property, such as jewelry, inappropriately.
- Markedly depressed patients who suddenly seem "better" may have made a decision to kill themselves. They feel relieved by deciding to do so and thereby take some action. The nurse may discover that they have telephoned others to say good-bye.
- People who are suicidal may be unable to articulate their feelings, may feel unheard, or may know no other way to call attention to themselves and the situation.
- If a patient admits to being suicidal, it is crucial to determine the patient's plan, the potential means, and also the availability of immediate access to complete the plan.
- Does the patient have a plan?
- If so, what is it?
- Is the patient imminently at risk in the hospital?
  - Is the patient thinking of jumping from a high hospital window or of using a knife or other sharp instrument? For example, one man who had had open-heart surgery cut his neck with a small penknife in the middle of the night while he was on the recovery unit. He had hidden the knife under his pillow and had been despondent over the loss of his wife, who had died 6 months earlier.
  - Other patients may be thinking of shooting themselves, but they do not have a gun.

- Others may be thinking of taking a lethal overdose of medications by not swallowing medication given by the nurse and saving it; or by taking large amounts of drugs already in their possession.

DSM-IV-TR DIAGNOSES

These psychiatric diagnoses may be related to the suicidal act

- Bipolar disorder
- Major depressive disorder
- Noncompliance with treatment
- Schizophrenia
- Substance use disorders

NANDA NURSING DIAGNOSES

The nursing diagnoses that are directly related to the suicidal act include

- Risk for self-directed violence
- Hopelessness
- Noncompliance
- Self-mutilation
- Risk for self-mutilation

Other nursing diagnoses are relevant to each person's precipitating problems; for example, diagnoses might be related to the person's inability to cope, their grief, or overwhelming feelings of depression.

NURSING INTERVENTIONS

The following nursing interventions can be used with a patient who is actually or potentially suicidal.

- **Intervention:** Assess the patient's suicidal intent.
    - Ask the patient directly about suicidal thoughts.
    - Always take threats of suicide seriously and assess the imminent lethality potential.
    - Continually assess the patient's impulse control.

    Rationale: Once a correct assessment is made of the patient's suicidal ideation, steps can be taken to ensure the patient's safety.
- **Intervention:** Establish a therapeutic relationship with the patient.
    - Spend time with the patient.
    - Encourage expression of feelings and verbalization of thoughts.

    Rationale: The patient may experience an increase in self-esteem, feelings of safety, and feeling some relief from overwhelming thoughts and feelings if these interventions are implemented.
- **Intervention:** Create a safe environment by instituting safety precautions.
    - The patient should be visible, within eyesight of staff members, or checked often or monitored by using some system in which staff members are accountable for the patient's whereabouts.
    - The patient may need one-on-one care or monitoring whereby he or she is with a staff member, at arms length, and in full view at all times.
    - Medications should be taken in the presence of a nurse, and the patient should be checked for "cheeking" (not swallowing the pills, holding them in a corner of the mouth).
    - The patient's property should be examined, and any potentially dangerous objects (e.g., glass, razor, scissors, knives, belts) should be removed.

Rationale: Treatment can be sought or begun while the patient is protected from self-harm.

- **Intervention:** Provide nursing management for any possible sequelae from an unsuccessful suicide attempt (e.g., an aborted shooting, cutting, hanging, overdose, poisoning).

  Rationale: Emergency medical care needs to be instituted for life support.

- **Intervention:** Make a verbal behavioral contract with the patient, if appropriate.

  Rationale: The contract should include the expectation that the patient will not harm himself or herself and will seek out staff members to verbalize suicidal feelings. Most suicidal patients experience ambivalence and can be prompted into remaining safe by having them "give their word" to follow through on the safety contract.

- **Intervention:** Help the patient use effective coping methods.
  - Help the patient recognize unhealthy coping mechanisms.
  - Encourage the use of a problem-solving approach, with a focus on short-term resolution of the problem.

  Rationale: Suicidal patients often feel unable to see other ways out and need to build their way into the future.

- **Intervention:** Help the patient assess his or her strengths and weaknesses.
  - Help patients recognize actual resources, both personal and social, and potential ones not yet considered.

  Rationale: When coping methods are increased, solutions to some of life's problems can be attained.

- **Intervention:** If the patient is cognitively impaired, evaluate the patient's mental status and institute reality testing along with reorientation.

  Rationale: Patients can be protected from inadvertently and unintentionally harming themselves as a result of a thought disorder.

- **Intervention:** Notify and alert appropriate caregivers about the risk for suicide and the plan of care.

  Rationale: Appropriate communication to other caregivers and consistency in approach will be helpful.

- **Intervention:** Make referrals for immediate and long-term discharge needs.

  Rationale: The reason for the patient's suicidal ideation should be diagnosed and treated. The patient should be monitored continually until he or she is no longer suicidal.

SUMMARY

Suicide attempts and gestures must always be taken seriously and considered a call for help. The expected outcome when caring for patients who are suicidal is that they will not inflict physical self-injury and will develop adequate coping resources that are available and mobilized.

EXAM QUESTIONS

CHAPTER 5

Questions 25-31

25. According to the Centers for Disease Control and Prevention, suicide ranks as what number as the leading cause of death?

    a. 50th

    b. 75th

    c. 100th

    d. 11th

26. Which group has the highest suicide rate?

    a. Women age 45 and younger.

    b. White men age 85 and older.

    c. Patients with acute medical problems.

    d. Persons age 25 and older.

27. A suicide attempt is often precipitated by

    a. a telephone call.

    b. ingestion of a chemical substance.

    c. a major loss.

    d. a manic episode.

28. A risk factor to consider during a lethality assessment is the

    a. patient's education.

    b. patient's coping resources and suicide plan.

    c. patient's marital status and number of children.

    d. patient's physical endurance and future goals.

29. A myth about suicide is

    a. suicidal ideation is not inherited.

    b. suicidal patients are ambivalent about death.

    c. asking a patient directly about suicidal ideation will encourage him to make a suicide attempt.

    d. suicidal patients rarely call for help after a suicide attempt.

30. A psychiatric diagnosis that may be related to the suicidal act is

    a. major depressive disorder.

    b. substance dependence.

    c. attention-deficit disorder.

    d. generalized anxiety disorder.

31. The most important nursing intervention when working with a suicidal patient is to

    a. provide support and reassurance.

    b. teach stress management.

    c. create a safe environment.

    d. change the patient's wound dressing.

CHAPTER 6

NURSING MANAGEMENT OF THE PSYCHOTIC PATIENT

CHAPTER OBJECTIVE

After completing this chapter, the reader will be able to recognize psychosis in a patient and intervene appropriately.

LEARNING OBJECTIVES

After studying this chapter, the reader will be able to

1. define psychosis, perceptions, hallucinations, and delusions.
2. discuss the causative factors associated with psychosis.
3. indicate the signs and symptoms of psychosis.
4. list NANDA nursing and *DSM-IV-TR* diagnoses related to psychosis.
5. identify nursing interventions that can be used for a patient who is psychotic.

BACKGROUND

The most severe signs and symptoms of psychosis are the aberrant behaviors that many people label as "crazy." Persons who are experiencing hallucinations and suffering from delusions constitute a fair percentage of patients on psychiatric wards. Patients who are psychotic often are feared and shunned when personnel who are not knowledgeable mental health professionals care for them. Generally, psychotic persons are not dangerous; however, because their thinking is irrational, their behavior may be also irrational and can, therefore, be unpredictable.

Usually, a general hospital nurse can expect to work with patients who are acutely and briefly psychotic because of some organic cause. Additionally, patients who have schizophrenia or other psychotic illnesses sometimes require treatment in general hospitals and need thoughtful, specialized and thoughtful nursing care for their medical and psychiatric problems.

DEFINITIONS

Cognitive abilities: A person's abilities of thinking, including the ability to reason, to make inferences, and to understand.

Delusion: A false belief as a manifestation of a thought disorder.

Hallucination: A sensory perception that occurs without external stimulation of the relevant sensory organ. As a manifestation of a thought disorder, these are usually auditory. They may be visual, tactile, gustatory, or olfactory, but these are more often a manifestation of an organic disorder.

Perceptions: Identification and initial interpretation of a stimulus based on information received through the five senses.

Psychosis: A disordered state of thinking, often characterized by hallucinations or delusions.

Schizophrenia: A severe and persistent mental illness characterized by disordered thinking, impaired social and vocational functioning; the most disabling of the mental illnesses.

PREVALENCE

People may be psychotic for a variety of medical and psychiatric reasons. These include brain disorders, reactions to some medications, and biochemical disturbances. Schizophrenia occurs worldwide. Approximately, 1 in 100 people in the United States has schizophrenia. The vast majority of the patients with schizophrenia have it for their lifetime (APA, 2000; WFFSAAD, 2003).

CAUSATIVE FACTORS

A psychosis may be acute or chronic. It may be the sequela of organic or functional disorders (a condition that fails to reveal any evidence of physiologic or structural abnormalities). As previously mentioned, in the general hospital psychoses associated with psychiatric illness are seen less often than those associated with medical or organic illnesses.

Psychiatric Causes

- *Schizophrenia:* Schizophrenia is a disorder with multiple psychological impairments that commonly include psychosis (Table 6-1).
- *Mood disorders:* Persons with severe depression and some with bipolar affective illness may experience psychotic thinking.
- *Personality disorders:* Some persons who have a severe disturbance of personality may have episodes of disordered thinking and exhibit symptoms of psychosis.
- *Crisis:* Some persons in the midst of a crisis have disordered thought processes and may become transiently psychotic.
- *Sensory deprived or overstimulated:* Patients who are sensory deprived or over-stimulated have an increase in stress and thus can become psychotic. Many hospital intensive care units (ICUs) use the terms ICU psychosis and ICU-itis. This condition is thought to be a result of simply being a patient in an ICU and experiencing an overabundance of noise, odors, and the physical procedures done by so many physicians, nurses, and technicians throughout the day and night.

Organic Causes

The organic causes of psychosis are more easily defined. Such psychoses are generally short term, unless they stem specifically from a chronic illness. The major types of causes are:

- *Brain dysfunction:* Either brain damage from an assault or trauma or a brain disorder associated with some disease or lesion can cause psychosis.

  Some patients with organic brain disorders, including patients with delirium or dementia, may become psychotic.

  High fevers, acute infections, and systemic illness can cause psychosis.
- *Toxic substances:* A toxic response to various substances and medications can induce psychosis.

  Some medications, such as levodopa, can cause psychosis.

  With others, such as steroids, withdrawal from the medication can cause psychosis.

  Drug abusers can become psychotic. For some drugs (such as with LSD, PCP, mescaline, and the hallucinogens), the cause of the psychosis is the drug's specific action.

  High doses of other drugs, such as crystal

TABLE 6-1: *DSM-IV-TR* MEDICAL DIAGNOSES RELATED TO SCHIZOPHRENIA

SCHIZOPHRENIA	ESSENTIAL FEATURES
Schizophrenia	Two or more of the following symptoms-lasting 1-month (or less than if successfully treated): Delusions; Hallucinations; Disorganized speech; Grossly disorganized or catatonic behavior; Negative symptoms, affective flattening, alogia, or avolition
Types of Schizophrenia	
Catatonic	Meets basic criteria for schizophrenia; Motoric immobility as evidenced by catalepsy (including waxy flexibility) or stupor; Excessive motor activity (that is apparently purposeless and not influenced by external stimuli); Extreme negativism or mutism; Peculiarities of voluntary movement as evidenced by posturing (voluntary assumption of inappropriate or bizarre postures), stereotyped movements, prominent mannerism, or prominent grimacing; Echolalia or echopraxia
Disorganized	Meets basic criteria for schizophrenia; Disorganized speech; Disorganized behavior; Flat or inappropriate affect
Paranoid	Meets the basic criteria for schizophrenia; Preoccupation with one or more delusions or frequent auditory hallucinations; Disorganized speech, disorganized or catatonic behavior, and flat or inappropriate affect not prominent
Residual	There is continuing evidence of the disturbance, as indicated by the presence of negative symptoms or two symptoms listed in Criteria A for schizophrenia; Present in an attenuated form (e.g., odd beliefs, unusual perceptual experiences); Absence of prominent delusions, hallucinations, disorganized speech, and grossly disorganized or catatonic
Schizoaffective disorder	Meets the basic criteria for schizophrenia; An uninterrupted period of illness during which, at some time, there is either a major depressive episode, a manic episode, or a mixed episode concurrent with symptoms that meet Criteria A for schizophrenia
Schizophreniform disorder	Meets the basic criteria for schizophrenia; An episode of the disorder lasts at least 1 month but less than 6 months
Undifferentiated type	Meets the basic criteria for schizophrenia; Criteria for paranoid, disorganized or catatonic type

Note. From *Schizophrenia and Other Psychotic Disorders. Diagnostic and Statistical Manual of Mental Disorders,* Fourth Edition, *Text Revision,* by the American Psychiatric Association. 2000, Washington, DC: American Psychiatric Association. Reprinted with permission.

methamphetamine, other amphetamines, cocaine, and crack, can induce psychoses.

Alcoholic delirium or delirium tremens, the severe sign of withdrawal from alcohol, may include psychosis.

As with any toxic or foreign substance, any specific drug can have an adverse effect on someone, either during the period of intoxication or in the withdrawal phase. These adverse effects may precipitate a psychotic episode.

SIGNS AND SYMPTOMS

The two most severe indications of psychosis are hallucinations and delusions.

Psychotic people may exhibit any number of strange and bizarre behaviors. Aside from these, the manner of communication can be indicative of their altered thinking. It is not only in the way people speak but also in the process and content of what that psychosis may be evident.

Hallucinations

All forms of hallucinations can vary in their severity; some are mild and some are severe. The amount of cognitive impairment that causes the hallucination or the functioning that results from hallucinations varies from person to person and may even be different in each episode for each person.

Hallucinations may take different forms

- *Auditory:* Hearing voices or noises that are not truly present is by far the most common form of hallucination. Examples include hearing a dead family member speak and hearing the voice of God or the devil.
- *Visual:* Seeing objects that are not there. Examples are seeing bats flying around the room and seeing bugs crawling on the wall.
- *Olfactory:* Smelling strange, different, or unique odors (generally the patient is preoccupied with them). Examples are foul body odors, animal odors, "the smell of disease," and some caustic chemical smell or odor.
- *Gustatory:* Having a bad (i.e., strange, perhaps foul and nauseating) taste in the mouth, sometimes associated with eating or drinking something. An example is drinking something that tastes like "poison or blood."
- *Tactile:* Having things feel strange to the touch or having strange bodily sensations (e.g., bugs crawling on the body); experiencing objects as feeling odd and different.

Delusions

Delusions are false beliefs that generally follow some theme

- *Grandeur:* An inflated belief in one's self-importance or believing that one is someone prominent (who may be dead or alive), such as Jesus Christ, God, Napoleon, or Joan of Arc.
- *Persecution:* A dreadful sense of being followed, pursued, or threatened by others in a harmful manner. A person might believe that the Federal Bureau of Investigation, the Central Intelligence Agency, or the Mafia "is out to get me."
- *Reference:* A belief that environmental events and situations or other persons' behavior has a special relationship to the patient, sometimes in a controlling manner. Examples are seeing two people holding hands as a message that the patient will never experience a love relationship and receiving coded messages from the television or radio.
- *Somatic delusion:* A false sense of how one's body is functioning. For example, a perfectly healthy woman "knows" that she is dying from cancer that is rampant in her body.

OTHER SIGNS AND SYMPTOMS

- *Inappropriate affect:* Note the appearance of the patient's face. Is the patient laughing at some tragic news or crying about something funny? Does the way the patient appear match the context of the situation and the content of their speech?
- *Regression:* Some patients with long psychiatric histories seem quite dependent and needy; they behave in a childlike manner.
- *Hyper-religiosity:* Some patients seem overly religious. They are involved fervently with the church, God, and the Bible, often to the exclusion of all else. Sometimes the religious persuasion is questionable, and the beliefs may seem to be of a delusional proportion to reality.
- *Concrete thinking:* The patient takes what other people say literally. People with schizophrenia or developmental retardation think in this primitive manner.
- *Looseness of associations:* The patient connects random thoughts and experiences in a loose and perhaps strange way that does not make much sense.
- *Strange mechanisms of speech:* Patients who are psychotic, especially those who are schizophrenic, may use odd patterns of speech. These include echolalia, repeating what another person says; neologisms, making up new words that have hidden meanings and then using the new words in the course of conversation thinking others understand them; and word salad, using a jumble of mixed-up words in a sentence.

ASSESSMENT

Nursing assessment of the psychotic patient should include a mental status examination. During your interview of the patient, you may elicit bizarre and strange remarks and behaviors. Observe the patient closely. Look for excessive signs of stress, tension, and agitation.

Patients who are hallucinating (seeing objects, hearing voices) or are delusional (having false beliefs) may:

- Look vacant.
- Be attentive to something that is not obvious to you.
- Appear watchful and apprehensive.
- Seem quite internally preoccupied or distractible.
- Seem to have difficulty understanding you and following your conversation.
- Mumble or talk to themselves.
- Use socially unacceptable speech, such as curses and erratic tones of voice.

Document the evidence of psychotic communication and thinking. Describe the exact nature of the patient's psychosis. Document the patient's responses by citing direct quotes from the patient and giving specifics of any unusual mannerisms, dress, or behaviors.

Check the patient's history for previous psychiatric disorders, and report the psychosis to the patient's physician and related health care providers.

Once the cause of the patient's psychosis has been determined, treatment can begin, and planning for long-term care can be considered.

DSM-IV-TR DIAGNOSES

These psychiatric diagnoses may be related to the psychotic patient

- Mood disorder with psychotic features
- Psychotic disorders due to a general medical condition
- Schizophrenia and other psychotic disorders
- Substance-related disorders

NANDA NURSING DIAGNOSES

The following NANDA nursing diagnoses may be relevant to the psychotic patient

- Impaired verbal communication
- Ineffective coping
- Disturbed sensory perception
- Disturbed thought processes
- Risk for other-directed violence
- Risk for self-directed violence

NURSING INTERVENTIONS

The following nursing interventions can be used for patients who are psychotic

- **Intervention:** Establish rapport and a trusting relationship.
  - Make brief but frequent contacts with the patient.
  - Approach the patient with acceptance and a nonthreatening manner.

  Rationale: These measures provide support and reassurance.
- **Intervention:** Provide a safe environment.
  - Check the patient's potential for self-harm or harm to others.
  - Observe the patient often.
  - Command hallucinations, voices that tell a person to harm himself or herself, are extremely dangerous to the patient's safety.
  - Persons who are delusional and feel persecuted may act out violently, irrationally, and impulsively toward others.

  Rationale: Psychotic patients can be distraught enough to attempt suicide or may assault others.
- **Intervention:** Decrease stimulation.

  Rationale: If the patient is overly excited or responding to a great deal of anxiety, creating a more relaxing, restful, and calming atmosphere may decrease the entire episode or the intensity of the psychosis.
- **Intervention:** Do not argue with psychotic patients.
  - Let them know you believe they are in fact reporting the truth as they know it.
  - Tell them the reality from your perspective.
  - Remind them of time, place, and person.
  - You may want to say, "I know you are fearful of being harmed by aliens, but there is no evidence of their presence here now," or "I don't see any spiders. I believe that you do. Let us talk about how we can help you to feel safe."

  Rationale: These approaches provide reality orientation and a sense of safety.
- **Intervention:** Make sure you understand what the patient means.
  - Ask questions.
  - Summarize what you think has been said.

  Rationale: Misinterpretation can occur easily.
- **Intervention:** Help patients determine when and why they become anxious.
  - Use problem solving with them to find ways to cope with anxiety.
  - Do this before or after, not during, a psychotic episode.

  Rationale: Anxiety can stimulate signs and symptoms of psychosis.
- **Intervention:** Use physical contact cautiously.

  Rationale: Patients who believe they are being persecuted or who are irrational may misinterpret physical contact and overreact.
- **Intervention:** Communicate assessments to the physician.

Rationale: The physician most likely will order an antipsychotic medication to alleviate the signs and symptoms of psychosis.

- **Intervention:** Administer psychopharmacologic medications when necessary as directed by a physician.

  Rationale: These medications are used to manage the symptoms of schizophrenia, organic brain syndrome with psychosis, depressive episode with psychotic features and substance-related disorders.

CASE STUDY

A 47-year-old man was admitted to the hospital 3 weeks ago for evaluation of a possible brain tumor or aneurysm. Before admission, he was markedly healthy. His one sign, which prompted him to seek the care of a physician, was a drooping eyelid. The droop had increased slowly over the course of 1 week, and the lid had closed fully on the 7th day.

After an extensive workup including computed tomography, brain scans, electroencephalography, magnetic resonance imaging, and numerous radiographic studies and hematologic tests, a diagnosis of Burkitt's lymphoma, a rare illness, was made. The patient was scheduled for neurosurgery to implant a shunt that would allow chemotherapeutic agents to be administered directly into his brain.

This patient had no previous history of emotional problems, but throughout the course of his 3-week hospitalization had shown gradually increasing signs of anxiety about the eventual outcome of his illness.

The morning after the neurosurgery, the nurse notices that the patient is markedly agitated. He is gesturing with his arm and seems to be mumbling and whispering.

He says to the staff nurse, "Nurse, nurse, there's a conspiracy going on here. Did you know that? Dr. Jones and Dr. Black are playing with my head; they're doing some kind of mind games. I have been seeing things flying around the room all night. Are these hallucinations or what? Get Dr. Smith; he's the only good one left. I don't trust the rest. Hurry, hurry!" The patient seems to be about to pull out his IV line and jump out of the bed. As he is talking, his agitation is increasing.

Although the staff nurse is somewhat apprehensive, she does the following:

- *With a calm demeanor and using a low modulated voice, introduces herself and reminds the patient where he is and about his recent surgery.*
- *Assures the patient that she understands his beliefs and believes he is experiencing hallucinations. She tells him that hallucinations are understandable because of his stress over the surgery and severe illness and says that she does not see things flying around the room.*
- *Indicates to another staff member that she might need some help in restraining this patient for the patient's safety.*
- *Reports the patient's psychosis and agitation to his physicians.*
- *Monitors the patient's behaviors often. Stays with him and does an assessment by using a mini-mental status examination.*
- *Frequently orients the patient and does reality tests.*
- *Clearly and concisely explains all procedures necessary.*
- *This man's psychosis may have stemmed from a variety of causes:*

  His neurosurgery

  His brain disease

  His prolonged hospitalization with the multiple, some invasive, diagnostic procedures

  Some of his medications

Chances are good that this episode will be brief and transient. Most likely, the patient will return to his nonpsychotic state within hours once appropriate treatment is started.

EXAM QUESTIONS

CHAPTER 6

Questions 32-36

32. The term psychosis is
    a. smelling things.
    b. an inflated belief in oneself.
    c. having hallucinations or delusions or both.
    d. a major tranquilizer.

33. A psychiatric cause associated with psychosis is
    a. conduct disorder.
    b. schizophrenia.
    c. separation anxiety disorder.
    d. attention-deficit/hyperactivity disorder.

34. If a patient hears voices or noises that are not truly present, he is experiencing a type of hallucination called
    a. olfactory.
    b. gustatory.
    c. auditory.
    d. tactile.

35. A nursing diagnosis for disturbed thought processes is associated with
    a. cognitive dissonance.
    b. psychiatric dysfunction.
    c. psychosis.
    d. psychoanalysis.

36. One of the most important assessments of a psychotic patient is
    a. checking the patient's potential for self-harm or harm to others.
    b. establishing a therapeutic relationship.
    c. documenting evidence of psychotic communication.
    d. getting a full medical history.

CHAPTER 7

NURSING MANAGEMENT OF THE PATIENT WITH SUBSTANCE-RELATED DISORDERS

CHAPTER OBJECTIVE

After completing this chapter, the reader will be able to identify substance-related disorders and discuss nursing interventions that may be useful in caring for a patient with a disorder of this type.

LEARNING OBJECTIVES

After studying this chapter, the reader will be able to

1. discuss the theories of causation for alcoholism and other substance-related disorders.
2. identify early warning signs of alcoholism, signs and symptoms of alcohol withdrawal, and treatments used for detoxification and rehabilitation.
3. discuss the signs, symptoms, and treatment for amphetamine, cocaine, heroin, sedative, hypnotic, and anxiolytic intoxication and withdrawal, and long-term recovery for these states.
4. recognize the relevant NANDA nursing diagnoses and *DSM-IV-TR* diagnoses related to substance use and abuse.

OVERVIEW

Cultural traditions surround the use of alcohol in family, religious, and social settings. There are marked differences in the quantity, frequency, and patterning of alcohol consumption in the countries of the world. In the United States 66-90% of adults have consumed alcohol. Amphetamine is abused throughout all levels of society and is more common among younger adults. Cannabinoids are the most widely used illicit psychoactive substance used in the United States. The prevalence of cocaine use in the United States has fluctuated over the years (*DSM-IV-TR*, 2000)

In every health care setting, nurses come in contact with patients who have substance abuse and dependency problems. For patients who abuse drugs or are chemically dependent, the manner in which a nurse cares for them is important. Those who work in emergency departments are familiar with the substance abuser as a patient. In some parts of the United States, cocaine, crack, and PCP have brought increased violence into the emergency department. Patients with drug-related problems are seen on medical-surgical and even maternity units, where mothers who are drug-addicted give birth to drug-addicted neonates.

The nurse may be the patient's first contact with a health care provider. The nurse has an opportunity to intervene by providing assessment, corroboration, referral, and collaboration with the patient and the members of the patient's health care team and family.

NURSING ATTITUDES

The nurse can potentially make an impact on or influence the resistance of patients who are chemically dependent. It is essential for nurses to examine their own attitudes and beliefs about addicts and addiction before working with chemically dependent patients. For example, it is helpful when nurses understand and believe that addiction is an illness rather than a moral weakness.

DEFINITIONS OF TERMS

Clarification of concepts/terms associated with chemical dependence is necessary to begin to understand the illness.

Alcoholism: A disorder characterized by out-of-control consumption of alcohol, resulting in biological, social, and vocational functional impairment.

Abuse: The continued use of substances (alcohol and other drugs) over a prolonged period of time even after problems occur.

Delirium: A disordered mental status characterized by confusion, agitation, and hallucinations.

Delirium tremens: A disordered mental state, or delirium, that occurs during withdrawal from alcohol.

Dependence: A cluster of cognitive, behavioral, and physiological symptoms indicating that the individual continues use of the substance despite significant substance-related problems (*DSM-IV-TR*, 2000).

Habit: The constant desire for, and use of, a substance in the absence of a physical dependence, although a psychological dependence may be present.

Organic delusional disorder: An organic disorder characterized by alteration in thought processes in which the person affected has false beliefs.

Organic hallucinosis: An organic disorder characterized by alteration in thought processes in which the person affected has hallucinations.

Substance: A drug of abuse, a medication, or a toxin.

Tolerance: The need for greatly increased amounts of the substance to achieve intoxication (or desired effect) or a markedly diminished effect with continued use of the same amount of the substance (*DSM-IV-TR*, 2000).

Withdrawal: A maladaptive behavioral change, with physiological and cognitive concomitants, that occurs when blood or tissue concentrations of a substance decline in an individual who had maintained prolonged heavy use of the substance (*DSM-IV-TR*, 2000).

THEORIES OF CAUSATION

Alcoholism

At this time, no single definitive cause of alcoholism is known. Nevertheless, many aspects of alcoholism are well known, including common problems and issues for possible causation. Early warning signs and generalities are earmarks of potential problems. A combination of physical, psychological, and social factors seems logical, in the context of each alcoholic's personal life.

Physical factors

- Because a high rate of alcoholism is seen in families, a genetic link cannot be ruled out. Another theory is that an endocrine dysfunction may cause a desire or a predisposition for alcohol.
- The allergy theory proposes that in some persons the body has an allergic response to alcohol.
- A nutritional theory claims that some deficiencies may cause a craving for alcohol.

Psychological factors

- Psychological factors include extreme dependence, needing "oral" gratification, and drinking for relief of tension.

Social factors

- Social factors include excessive drinking as a result of patterns found in the family and being "socialized" to drink at a young age. In addition, some cultural and ethnic groups drink more than others do, and more men than women are alcoholics, although the number of women with alcoholism is increasing.

Substance Abuse

Like alcoholism, substance abuse seems to have no single known causative factor. It seems to manifest itself in a person who is experiencing a combination of biological, psychological, and social phenomena. Our society has been medically and commercially socialized to "pop" pills: "Have a headache, toothache? Take an aspirin, Tylenol, Motrin." Children are raised in a comfortable-with-pills atmosphere.

Young people often begin abusing substances because of peer pressure. The vulnerable preteen time and adolescence experienced by some lead to drug-taking behaviors to be part of the crowd and to fit in. Some adolescents may be rebelling against their parents, other authority figures, and society itself. Others may be looking for an escape from their perceived problems and feelings of depression. These children are looking for a way out of their present reality.

The 1960s saw many persons experiencing drug-seeking moods and mind-altering states. Once substances of abuse are tried, different variables seem to come into play that determine whether or not the person develops a drug abuse problem. The user's place in society, self-esteem and self-concept, age, peers, finances, lifestyle, personality characteristics, and other physical and emotional problems intermingle. Abuse of prescription medicines may start with a defined ailment. However, use can quickly become a convoluted problem, with increasing reliance on some drugs such as painkillers.

In view of the different drugs readily available, it is no surprise that polysubstance abuse (abusing more than one drug at a time) has become a problem. Although all the drugs used are associated with some degree of psychological dependence, some are physically addicting. They cause a craving and tolerance, and discontinuing them causes a great deal of physical discomfort, so much so that the need for the drug is heightened. Heroin addiction is an example of this phenomenon.

Many researchers are dissatisfied with the inconclusiveness of psychosocial theories of drug dependence and are focusing their attention on biochemical factors related to drug use. Nothing conclusive has been proven yet.

SUBSTANCE-RELATED DISORDERS

Alcohol

Alcohol is the most pervasive substance of abuse of all toxic chemicals. It is a liquid contrary to popular belief, is not a stimulant but that acts as a CNS depressant. Early signs and symptoms of intoxication, such as giddiness, talkativeness, loosening of inhibitions, and relaxation, seem socially appealing, but continued use can result in serious physiological, psychological, and social consequences.

An assessment should be made of the person's dependence on alcohol and the possible ensuring sequelae of social problems, such as marital, work-related, or legal (e.g., drunk driving or arrests for assault) which follow. Physical illnesses such as liver, GI, and neurologic problems, and recurrent injury can provide clues to alcoholism. Emotional problems, such as depression, insomnia, and irritability, can be indications of alcohol abuse.

A description of alcohol use includes the amount and frequency of alcohol consumption and any evidence of the presence of alcohol withdrawal symptoms.

Alcohol Effects

Alcohol acts differently in each person. Some of the effects are related to each person's absorption time which can be affected by variables such as the following:

- Amount of alcohol consumed
- How fast the alcoholic drinks follow each other
- The person's body weight, height, and general size
- Presence or absence of food in the stomach
- Stomach emptying time, metabolic rate
- Presence of progressive psychological and physical dependence on alcohol has occurred progressively. Alcoholics are unable to stop drinking and often drink to excess.

Alcohol Intoxication

People who are intoxicated are usually not too difficult to recognize. After a recent ingestion of alcohol, they generally have some or all of the following:

- Odor of alcohol on the breath
- Emotional lability, ranging from euphoria to hostility
- Slurred speech
- Incoordination and ataxia
- Nystagmus
- Impaired judgment
- Decreased inhibitions, aggressiveness, increased sexual impulses
- Memory or attention impairment
- Stupor or coma

Warning Signs of Alcoholism

The warning signs of alcoholism include the following:

- A loss of control over drinking: sneaking drinks, drinking until unconscious, drinking in the morning.
- Social and occupational problems: arguing about drinking with spouse and other family members, missing work because of drinking or being hung over, not keeping engagements, becoming unreliable.
- Blackout episodes: times when the person is functioning but has no recall for events.
- Legal complications: convicted of driving under the influence of alcohol.

Alcohol Abuse

Alcohol abuse refers to patterns of alcohol use with the continuation of drinking despite marital discord, job threats, and legal and physical problems. An example of someone who abuses alcohol is a person who continues to drink and drive, despite repeated convictions for driving under the influence of alcohol (*DSM-IV-TR*, 2000).

Alcohol Dependence

Alcohol dependence is diagnosed on the basis of persistence, craving, and continual use and generally is thought to include a withdrawal syndrome.

The progressive course of alcoholism can range from mild signs and symptoms of hangover, missing or being late to work, and some marital discord to total craving and dependence on alcohol. Alcohol dependence may be associated with a complete breakdown in the family, a loss of job, poor health, and signs and symptoms of withdrawal.

Alcohol Addiction

Alcohol addiction knows no barriers. Men, women, teenagers, elderly people, and even young children have experienced problems with alcoholism. Numerous medical complications are associated with alcohol addiction, and patients in the general hospital, who are there for any number of reasons, also can be in an early or later stage of alcohol-related disease. Because denial is such a strong component of alcoholism, many alcoholics refuse to acknowledge their addiction.

Physical Complications Associated with Alcoholism

Alcoholism is a progressive disease, which can be fatal. A number of physiologic problems and potential diseases are related to excessive drinking. Table 7-1 gives some of the physical complications associated with alcoholism. Patients who have these problems may show up first in the general hospital for treatment of the alcohol-related problem or because of other health-related issues. The presence of these problems may provide clues to a patient's covert alcoholism.

Alcohol Withdrawal

In a general hospital setting, a patient can be an unknown alcoholic and be receiving treatment for a problem that might be related or unrelated to their alcoholism. Because patients usually have to suddenly cease drinking upon admission, nurses must be aware of the signs and symptoms of alcohol withdrawal. These include the following:

- Autonomic hyperactivity
- Increased in hand tremors
- Tachycardia
- Psychomotor agitation
- Anxiety
- Nausea
- Vomiting
- Insomnia
- Grand mal seizures
- Transient, visual, tactile, or auditory hallucinations or illusions
- Delirium tremens

Withdrawal from alcohol generally occurs 24-72 hours after the last drink was taken. During withdrawal, the patient's health progressively dete-

TABLE 7-1: ALCOHOL-RELATED PHYSICAL COMPLICATIONS

System or Organs Involved	Complication
Brain, neurologic	Peripheral polyneuritis Wernicke-Korsakoff syndrome (disorientation, delirium, confusion, confabulation, ocular impairment; a progressive disorder that requires thiamine replacement)
Liver, pancreas	Alcoholic hepatitis Liver failure Pancreatitis
Muscle	Myopathy
Cardiopulmonary	Enlarged heart Susceptibility to infections Pneumonia
Gastrointestinal	Gastric distress Ulcers Nutritional imbalance
Hematologic	Anemia

riorates. Potential complications of alcohol withdrawal include the following:

- Aspiration pneumonia
- Peripheral vascular collapse
- Hyperthermia
- Infection
- Myocardial infarction
- Self-inflicted trauma, purposeful or accidental
- Death, because of one of the other complications

Treatment for delirium tremens (DTs)

The immediate treatment for present or impending delirium tremens is pharmacologic. A minor tranquilizer, usually a benzodiazepine such as Librium (chlordiazepoxide) or Ativan® (lorazepam), is used. The CNS depressant action of the drug helps minimize progression of the withdrawal. The benzodiazepine then can be titrated down gradually to the lowest effective dose until the patient is no longer at risk for serious sequelae of withdrawal. Eventually the medication can be discontinued.

Other problems to be considered are the patient's nutritional status, including fluid and electrolyte balance and levels of vitamins, thiamine, and magnesium. The potential for trauma or self-harm should be addressed as appropriate. Obviously, any imminent crisis (e.g., circulatory or respiratory collapse) must be attended to immediately.

***DSM-IV-TR* Diagnoses**

DSM-IV-TR diagnoses related to alcoholism include the following:

- Alcohol intoxication delirium
- Alcohol withdrawal delirium
- Alcohol-induced persisting amnestic disorder
- Alcohol-induced psychotic disorder
- Alcohol-induced persisting dementia
- Alcohol-induced psychotic disorder, with hallucinations
- Alcohol-induced psychotic disorder, with delusions
- Alcohol withdrawal
- Alcohol-induced anxiety disorder, mood disorder, sexual dysfunction, or sleep disorder

Treatments for Alcoholism

When the immediate effects of alcohol withdrawal are subsiding, the ongoing treatment for alcoholism as the primary disease problem needs to be considered. Most treatment programs in the United States are based on the idea of the "recovering" alcoholic. These programs advocate taking one day at a time, accepting the idea that the temptation to drink is ever-present in our society, and that abstinence is the only way to maintain sobriety.

A variety of treatment options are available. Inpatient programs are found in general hospitals, psychiatric hospitals, residential treatment facilities, and group homes. Outpatient treatment can be privately based or through the auspices of clinics, hospitals, or other public facilities. Of all of the outpatient programs, Alcoholics Anonymous (AA) is the most well known and widely used of the 12-step programs. It is free, anonymous, and supportive. Since the 1940s, it has been a growing, popular, and respected self-help program.

Public and private outpatient programs are available through clinics and private practitioners in a variety of disciplines, including physicians, nurses, social workers, psychologists, and drug and alcohol counselors. These programs may be group or individual oriented. Some offer residential treatment and then outpatient follow-up care.

Use of medications beyond the withdrawal period has been effective. Antabuse® (disulfiram) is used as an alcohol antagonist. Some patients, who cannot achieve sobriety independently, find that taking Antabuse® is enough of a deterrent to maintain abstinence. However, the benefits of this treatment are eliminated if the patient has no motivation for taking the antagonist.

Because the causes of alcoholism differ from person to person, a wide range of treatment approaches are effective. Self-help groups other than AA are available, including family and marital therapy (which can be an important adjunct as well), individual therapy, education programs, behavioral therapy, and aversion therapy.

Each person's situation, general health, emotional problems, amount of alcoholic disease, and life circumstances should be considered when recommendations for treatment are made. It may be preferable for the alcoholic to be an inpatient for a while removed from the pressures and commitments of everyday life in a place where treatment can be intensive. Conversely, being an inpatient may jeopardize a person's job, family, or social situation, and thus, beginning treatment as an outpatient might be a better option.

The trend in alcohol treatment is a multisystem effort. Programs include many different approaches. Usually a patient's treatment plan includes the following:

- Individual counseling
- Group therapy
- Daily educational meeting
- Family therapy
- Occupational therapy or vocational rehabilitation
- Recreational therapy
- Psychopharmacologic therapy

The increasing problem of alcoholism and the increased attention given to it by the medical community and the media have brought the "secret" of widespread abuse of alcohol out in the open. Treatment options are widely available to all who are comfortable in admitting they are alcoholics and seek help.

Other Substance-Related Disorders

Substance abuse has existed for centuries. Stories have been told of opium dens, mescaline dreams, and herbs and spirits used for changing one's level of consciousness and awareness and for enhancing mood. The drug of choice has varied, depending on the time and the country. At times, some drugs were legal and others were illegal (e.g., alcohol and cocaine).

In addition to alcohol, heroin has long been a substance of abuse. In the 1960s, marijuana, LSD, and other psychedelic drugs were the popular drugs of choice. "Downers" (barbiturates and tranquilizers) and the abuse of prescribed medicine followed. In the 1970s, "uppers" came to the forefront, along with PCP. The 1980s brought the cocaine crisis, including crack and crystal methamphetamine (crystal meth). All the previous drug problems continued as well.

Today, the problem of drug abuse has reached epidemic proportions. The issue of drug abuse persists and use of crack cocaine is particularly dangerous because its users often turn to violent crimes to support their habit. Any patient who is addicted to one or more substances and is currently hospitalized is at risk for withdrawal.

Amphetamine or Amphetamine-Like-Related Disorders

Amphetamines are CNS stimulants. They and other stimulants are used to treat obesity, attention deficit/hyperactivity disorder, and narcolepsy. However, they are generally avoided medically because of their high potential for abuse.

Amphetamine abuse signs and symptoms are as follows:

- Euphoria
- Hyperalertness
- Anorexia
- Increased pulse rate
- Increased blood pressure

- Insomnia
- Excessive talkativeness

Amphetamine withdrawal develops within a few hours to several days after cessation (or reduction) of amphetamine use that has been heavy or prolonged. The following signs and symptoms of amphetamine withdrawal include (*DSM-IV-TR*, 2000):

- Dysphoric mood
- Fatigue
- Vivid, unpleasant dreams
- Insomnia or hypersomnia
- Increased appetite
- Psychomotor retardation or agitation

Cannabis

Marijuana and hashish generally produce a state of mild euphoria and relaxation. These illegal drugs are smoked in a "joint" (a home-rolled cigarette) or through a pipe. Hallucinations can occur with high doses. Lack of motivation and possible irreversible brain damage has been of concern in adolescents who smoke marijuana.

Cannabis intoxication includes the following signs and symptoms (*DSM-IV-TR*, 2000):

- Maladaptive behavior or psychological changes, for example, impaired motor coordination, euphoria, anxiety, impaired judgment
- Conjunctival injection
- Increased appetite
- Dry mouth
- Tachycardia

Cocaine

Cocaine seems to have been the scourge of the 1980s. When cocaine abuse first became widespread, it was considered a white-collar problem. The drug was expensive, and initially addiction and withdrawal problems were not seen. A fast-acting but short-lasting CNS stimulant, cocaine produces a rush of euphoria. The popularity of "coke," as it is commonly known, has continued and spread. The drug has found its way into poorer communities as crack cocaine, a cheaper, less pure, and smokable form of cocaine. Cocaine addiction has increased, and a withdrawal syndrome is now recognized.

The signs and symptoms of cocaine overdose include the following:

- Panic level of anxiety
- Increased pulse rate
- Increased blood pressure
- Dilated pupils
- Severe perspiration
- Syncope
- Seizures
- Episodes of delusions, paranoia, hallucinations, and mania
- Death, usually as a result of cardiac or respiratory failure

The signs and symptoms of cocaine withdrawal include the following (APA, 2000):

- Dysphoric mood
- Vivid, unpleasant dreams
- Fatigue
- Hypersomnia or insomnia
- Psychomotor retardation or agitation
- Increased appetite

Hallucinogens

The hallucinogens LSD, PCP, and mescaline are drugs that alter the user's sense of reality and consciousness. They cause a distorted sense of energy and excitement, and hallucinations and other perceptual changes may occur. LSD was popularized as "acid" in the hippie era of the 1960s. In the 1970s, PCP or angel dust was more common. Violent side effects are associated with the use of PCP. Users can become quite paranoid and delusional and act out impulsively. Personnel in the emergency department often have been assaulted while attempting to administer care to such patients.

Inhalants

Sniffing glue or inhaling other substances such as paint, paint thinner, gasoline, or even white-out (Liquid Paper) is a less common problem than other forms of drug abuse. Children and preteens are more apt than people in other age groups to use inhalants, probably because the substances are cheap and readily available. Inhalants and some other substances are seen as a "cheap high" in this school-age group and may cause not only social and school problems but also respiratory and neurological damage.

Opioids

Heroin, methadone, and narcotics such as morphine and Demerol® (meperidine) have long been known for their addictive properties and their definite and severe withdrawal patterns. Abused for their euphoric properties, these drugs also produce pain relief, apathy, and impaired judgment. Heroin addicts seem to be seeking release from daily woes.

The signs and symptoms of heroin overdose are as follows:

- Decreased respirations
- Pinpoint pupils
- Pale, cool, clammy skin with cyanotic tinge
- Needle tracks (marks) on the arms and legs or in areas of hidden veins
- Cardiac dysrhythmias
- Clouded consciousness, semicomatose states, coma
- Pulmonary edema
- Shock
- Death as a result of respiratory failure or cerebral edema

The signs and symptoms of withdrawal from opioids are as follows (APA, 2002):

- Dysphoric mood
- Nausea, vomiting
- Muscle aches
- Lacrimation or rhinorrhea
- Pupillary dilation, piloerection, or sweating
- Diarrhea
- Yawning
- Fever
- Insomnia

Sedatives, Hypnotics, and Anxiolytics

Sedatives, hypnotics, and anxiolytics are a group of tranquilizing drugs that cause quiescence, relaxation, and a decrease in tension and anxiety. Still prescribed medically and valuable for their beneficial effects, these drugs are highly misused and abused. Tolerance often develops, causing the need for increases in doses and frequency of use. If outright addiction does not occur, habituation and dependence are common.

The signs and symptoms of abuse and overdose of these drugs are as follows:

- Craving and tolerance
- Ataxia
- Irritable mood
- Slurred speech
- Sustained nystagmus
- Slowed reactions
- Lethargy
- Impaired judgment
- Confusion
- Disorientation
- Clouded consciousness
- Hypersomnia
- Coma

The signs and symptoms of withdrawal from sedatives, hypnotics, or anxiolytics are as follows (APA, 2000):

- Autonomic hyperactivity

- Increased hand tremors
- Insomnia
- Nausea, vomiting
- Transient visual, tactile, or auditory hallucinations
- Psychomotor agitation
- Anxiety
- Grand mal seizures

DSM-IV-TR DIAGNOSES

The groups of substances of abuse other than alcohol that are listed in *DSM-IV-TR* for both substance abuse and dependence include the following:

- Amphetamine withdrawal
- Cocaine withdrawal
- Opioid withdrawal
- Sedative, hypnotic, or anxiolytic withdrawal
- Amphetamine-induced psychotic disorder, with delusions or hallucinations
- Cannabis-induced psychotic disorder, with delusions or hallucinations
- Hallucinogen-induced psychotic disorder, with delusions or hallucinations
- Inhalant-induced psychotic disorder, with delusions or hallucinations
- Opioid-induced psychotic disorder, with delusions or hallucinations
- Phencyclidine-induced psychotic disorder, with delusions or hallucinations
- Sedative, hypnotic, or anxiolytic-induced psychotic disorder, with delusions or hallucinations
- Amphetamine intoxication delirium
- Cannabis intoxication delirium
- Cocaine intoxication delirium
- Hallucinogen intoxication delirium
- Inhalant intoxication delirium
- Opioid intoxication delirium
- Phencyclidine intoxication delirium
- Sedative, hypnotic, or anxiolytic intoxication delirium
- Substance-induced persisting dementia
- Sedative, hypnotic, or anxiolytic-induced persisting dementia
- Amphetamine-induced mood disorder, or anxiety disorder, sexual dysfunction, sleep disorder, or intoxication
- Cocaine-induced mood disorder, or anxiety disorder, sexual dysfunction, sleep disorder, or intoxication
- Hallucinogen-induced mood disorder, anxiety disorder, intoxication, perception disorder
- Inhalant-induced mood disorder, anxiety disorder, or intoxication
- Opioid-induced mood disorder, sexual dysfunction, sleep disorder, or intoxication
- Phencyclidine-induced mood disorder, anxiety disorder, or intoxication
- Sedative, hypnotic, or anxiolytic-induced mood disorder, anxiety disorder, sexual dysfunction, sleep disorder, or intoxication

NANDA NURSING DIAGNOSES

Numerous nursing diagnoses are possible in patients with an addiction problem. Patients generally have more than one of the following:

- Ineffective coping
- Compromised family coping
- Disabled family coping
- Ineffective denial
- Risk for Injury

- Chronic low self-esteem
- Disturbed sensory perception
- Disturbed thought processes
- Risk for other-directed violence
- Risk for self-directed violence
- Spiritual distress

Nursing diagnoses related to the potential physiologic sequelae of chemical dependency include the following:

- Activity intolerance
- Anxiety
- Imbalanced nutrition: less than body requirements
- Sleep deprivation
- Disturbed sleep pattern
- Diarrhea
- Bathing/hygiene self-care deficit
- Dressing/grooming self-care deficit
- Feeding self-care deficit
- Toileting self-care deficit
- Sexual dysfunction

TREATMENTS

Chemically dependent patients generally cannot achieve a drug-free lifestyle on their own. Because of the craving, cost, peer-group pressure, and increased need for the sometimes-illegal substances, continued abuse can cause serious damage in the user's life. Family, friends, job relationships, the community, and society at large may all be affected adversely.

As with alcoholism, treatment for a drug addiction should be self-motivated. Although outside forces — job, family, money, and health — can contribute to their reasoning, a chemically dependent person needs to want to quit. Along with the desire to become drug-free, help and support from others are extremely important.

The single predictive criterion for success or failure for all addicts is the level of motivation or lack of it. When motivation is high, a degree of recovery usually can be achieved.

Psychopharmacologic Therapy: Treatment For Withdrawal

Psychopharmacologic therapy is generally used for detoxification, in emergencies as antagonists, and for maintenance therapy (e.g., methadone for heroin addicts). Treatment should be individualized for each patient.

For some drugs of abuse associated with a physical withdrawal syndrome, psychopharmacologic treatment is available to help patients withdraw safely. Methadone (Dolophine®) is used successfully in withdrawal from heroin. Clonidine (Catapres®) is under investigation as a drug for withdrawal from opiates. Benzodiazepines (such as, Librium® and Valium®) are used sometimes for withdrawal from tranquilizers, cocaine, and amphetamines. Sometimes the drug of abuse is given in titrated-down doses until the drug is no longer necessary.

Inpatient and Residential Programs

For some patients, the need to be away from the drug-taking environment, place, or people is crucial to gaining freedom from a dependency. Others do better by maintaining their usual activities and find outpatient programs a better option.

In conjunction with an addict's general physical condition and state, the drug of abuse itself may be a factor in determining the best type of treatment. Some emergency or acute medical care may be needed, either for an overdose problem or for potential sequelae of withdrawal.

Hospitals, clinics, and private residential treatment facilities such as the Betty Ford Center in southern California, offer a wide range of services.

Outpatient programs, methadone clinics, and private practitioners also offer many services. These include the following:

- Individual therapy
- Group therapy, supportive and confrontative
- Family and marital counseling
- 12-step, anonymous groups
- Self-help recovery groups

Recovery

Recovery is not necessarily an all-or-nothing event. It is common for some relapses to occur. Therefore, patients must try again and again. Even though an addict may not remain drug-free, repeated failures should not be criticized. An attitude of acceptance and willingness to support an addict's attempts to attain and maintain a drug-free state should be fostered.

NURSING INTERVENTIONS

The following nursing interventions can be used for patients who are chemically dependent on alcohol or drugs:

- **Intervention:** Establish a therapeutic relationship with patients.

  Rationale: This will increase patients' trust in you and give them a feeling of safety and security.

- **Intervention:** Treat confused patients with dignity and respect.
  - Use their proper names.
  - Do not treat them as if they were children.

  Rationale: Being treated with dignity and respect increases patients' self-esteem and self-concept.

- **Intervention:** Be supportive of the patient.

  Rationale: Support from health care providers can help encourage freedom from substance abuse and increase the patient's low self-esteem.

- **Intervention:** Provide safety for the patient, from trauma and harm.

  Rationale: While under the influence of a substance, the patient cannot maintain his own safety needs.

- **Intervention:** Assess and continually monitor the patient for adverse medical sequelae of intoxication or withdrawal.

  Rationale: Some drugs may cause death as a result of cardiac or respiratory failure.

- **Intervention:** Assess and monitor the patient's mental status.

  Rationale: Mental status changes and fluctuates according to ingestion of the substance and the amount ingested.

- **Intervention:** Do reality testing with the patient.

  Rationale: Monitoring the fluctuations in the patient's level of awareness and comprehension enables you to make necessary changes in the care plan.

- **Intervention:** Encourage verbalization and exploration.

  Rationale: These measures help increase the patient's awareness of his or her problem areas.

- **Intervention:** Teach the patient about substance abuse, including the psychological, biological, and social ramifications.

  Rationale: Knowledge about substance abuse will help increase the patient's awareness of the potential for problems.

- **Intervention:** Assess available support and explore options.

  Rationale: Knowledge about available support and possible options can help patients recognize their potential strengths.

- **Intervention:** Provide role modeling.

  Rationale: Role modeling sets an example and shows patients that they can be drug-free.

- **Intervention:** Administer psychopharmacologic medications when necessary as directed by a physician.

  Rationale: Psychopharmacologic medications are generally used for detoxification, in emergencies as antagonists, and for maintenance therapy (e.g., methadone for heroin).

- **Intervention:** Teach and encourage the use of relaxation techniques.

  Rationale: Relaxation can provide relief from tension and decrease anxiety.

CASE STUDY

Mr. Collins is a 49-year-old man who works as a commodities trader and part-time real estate broker. Mr. Collins was admitted, through the emergency department, to a cardiac unit to have his status monitored after an episode of crushing chest pain with evidence of valve collapse. He was awaiting test results on his cardiac status to determine his need and suitability for bypass surgery.

On his first day on the unit, he appeared tense, nervous, and jittery. Although anxiety would be an appropriate response in his situation, Mr. Collin's primary nurse felt his agitation was more than what would be considered appropriate to the situation.

His primary nurse noticed that he was anxious, diaphoretic, tremulous, and sleepless. He had a rapid pulse, high blood pressure, an elevated body temperature, and loss of appetite. Although some of these signs and symptoms were attributable to his cardiac condition and his concern about it, Mr. Collins seemed to be in additional distress.

The primary nurse has 15 years of experience as a nurse. She planned her morning to include 10 minutes to sit and talk with Mr. Collins. She did not have the time to do a formal mental status examination, but she followed her intuition and asked the patient about his alcohol intake.

Mr. Collins admitted to excessive drinking. He not only drank a fifth of vodka every 2 nights but also drank every day at lunch, had 2-3 martinis each day, and had some Bloody Mary's 3-4 days a week "to get the day going right." He talked of feeling tremulous without drinking and said that by having a "nip" early in the day, he could keep up his pace.

Understanding that the primary nurse was concerned with his consumption, Mr. Collins quickly added, "At least I'm not snorting the white stuff through my nose like my coworkers. What can be harmful about drinking? I've always been a drinker; I can hold my liquor!"

Mr. Collins did need bypass surgery. He was transferred to a cardiac surgery unit. The primary nurse made sure to include his drinking history in the transfer report. Now in his third hospitalized day, Mr. Collins was at great risk for alcohol withdrawal. His surgery was successful, with a brief stay on a cardiac postoperative unit and then a transfer back to his original unit.

Once back on the unit, the primary nurse followed up by discussing his previous drinking behavior with him. This discussion was an important aspect of his discharge planning. She then conferred with his cardiologist. Although Mr. Collins had not as yet experienced terribly negative effects from his alcoholism, the serious and fragile nature of his medical condition precluded his ability to return to the same patterns and habits. In addition, his present drinking pattern would most likely get him into deeper trouble with alcoholism.

As part of the discharge planning, his cardiologist recommended that Mr. Collins participate in

AA meetings. This participation would help him come to terms with his drinking problem. Although Mr. Collins protested that he did not have a problem, his physician was firm in the recommendation and presented other outpatient options, a local chemical dependency program he knew of, and therapy with a psychiatrist colleague who worked in addiction medicine.

During Mr. Collins's cardiac rehabilitation on the cardiac unit, the primary nurse, who had established a rapport with him, helped him open up to her a little bit. She reviewed with him the dynamics and causes of his drinking, and the effect this behavior had on his general health and well-being.

This case is a typical example of a patient who is admitted to a general hospital with a primary disease or disorder that requires some medical or surgical intervention. In this situation, the patient's nurse can act as a primary resource to assess health problems and then collaborate with the patient and other health care providers to treat the secondary or underlying problem. Alcohol and other substance abuse problems can be addressed first by a nurse in this manner.

SUMMARY

Chemically dependent patients generally cannot achieve a drug-free lifestyle on their own. Treatment for a drug addiction should be self-motivated. The single predictive criterion for success or failure for all addicts is their level of motivation or lack of it. When motivation is high, a degree of recovery usually can be achieved.

EXAM QUESTIONS

CHAPTER 7

Questions 37-46

37. Peer pressure seems to contribute to

    a. drug abuse among some teenagers.
    b. early schizophrenic breakdown.
    c. withdrawal from drugs.
    d. the binge-purge cycle.

38. Drinking alcohol in the morning on a regular basis is considered

    a. social.
    b. an early warning sign of alcoholism.
    c. healthy by some physicians.
    d. helpful for tension relief.

39. Signs and symptoms of alcohol withdrawal are

    a. delirium tremens, anorexia, headache.
    b. fever, poor judgment, hypersomnia.
    c. tremors, tachycardia, insomnia.
    d. psychosomatic ills, tremors, bradycardia.

40. Potential complications of alcohol withdrawal are

    a. pulmonary edema and infection.
    b. anemia and ulcers.
    c. grand mal seizures and myopathy.
    d. aspiration pneumonia and myocardial infarction.

41. The two commonly used medications for alcohol withdrawal are

    a. chlordiazepoxide and pentobarbital.
    b. diazepam and triazolam.
    c. chlordiazepoxide and lorazepam.
    d. alcohol and phenobarbital.

42. Seizures, anxiety, and paranoia are signs and symptoms of

    a. psychotic depression.
    b. cocaine overdose.
    c. alcohol intoxication.
    d. dementia.

43. The signs or symptoms of amphetamine abuse are

    a. increased body temperature, increased blood pressure, increased pulse rate.
    b. increased pulse rate, decreased blood pressure, increased temperature.
    c. euphoria, anorexia, increased pulse rate.
    d. anorexia, increased blood pressure, increased body temperature.

44. The signs and symptoms of heroin overdose are

    a. decreased respirations, pinpoint pupils, pulmonary edema.
    b. depression, fatigue, pinpoint pupils.
    c. shock, increased blood pressure, insomnia.
    d. pinpoint pupils, decreased respiration, mouth sores.

45. Residential treatment facilities are used for patients who have

    a. depression.
    b. drug abuse problems.
    c. borderline personality disorders.
    d. organic brain syndromes.

46. The signs and symptoms of cocaine withdrawal are

    a. pinpoint pupils, decreased respirations, and nausea.
    b. slurred speech, increased appetite, and sweating.
    c. vivid unpleasant dreams, fatigue, and increased appetite.
    d. increased appetite, pinpoint pupils, and fever.

CHAPTER 8

NURSING MANAGEMENT OF THE CONFUSED PATIENT

CHAPTER OBJECTIVE

At the completing this chapter, the reader will be able to recognize the signs and symptoms of confusion in a patient and be able to apply sound principles of nursing care to confused patients.

LEARNING OBJECTIVES

After studying this chapter, the reader will be able to

1. describe delirium and dementia and recognize the differences between them.
2. discuss predisposing factors for varying types of confusion, including Alzheimer's disease.
3. list the NANDA nursing and *DSM-IV-TR* diagnoses related to caring for the confused patient.
4. identify nursing interventions that are helpful for the confused patient.

OVERVIEW

Patients who are confused pose special problems for the nurses in any area of nursing. The staffs of general hospital units and skilled nursing facilities need to be knowledgeable about the problem of confusion and the management of confused patients.

Whatever the causative factors, a confused, possibly brain-injured or brain-impaired patient is not thinking clearly and may misunderstand others as well as be misunderstood.

Patients with clouded consciousness, memory difficulties, and problems maintaining a reality base may behave bizarrely and not attend to basic functional needs. This condition may snowball and further impair the patient by adding a mood disorder, such as depression, that may contribute to an already increasing confusion.

DEFINITION OF TERMS

Delirium and dementia are commonly used terms. They are sometimes misidentified and confused with each other (Table 8-1).

Delirium: Delirium is a disordered mental status characterized by confusion, agitation, and hallucinations. Often delirium has a known precipitating event such as trauma, use of toxic substances, or a physical illness. It generally has an acute onset, is reversible, and lasts a short time. The waxing and waning of consciousness, which does not happen in dementia, characterize it.

Dementia: A dementia is usually more insidious. It may be chronic, slowly progressing over time, and with aging, perhaps becoming a permanent impairment. The specific cause may or may not be known or fully understood. However, dementia can be caused by an acute event such as a brain infarct.

Pseudodementia: Some elderly persons are prone to depression; possibly their depressive episode

TABLE 8-1: DIFFERENCES BETWEEN DELIRIUM AND DEMENTIA

FACTORS	Delirium	Dementia
Cause	Known precipitating event such as trauma, use of toxic substances, or a physical illness	Specific cause may or may not be known or fully understood; Can be caused by an acute event such as a brain infarct
Onset	Acute onset	Gradual onset More insidious
Course	Usually rapid course, but wide fluctuations; Usually reversible; Wide fluctuation	Chronic but continues to decline; Permanent impairment
Level of consciousness	Fluctuates May be difficult to arise to hyper-alert	Normal
Orientation	Disoriented; confused	Disoriented; confused
Affect	Fluctuating;	Labile Apathy in later stages
Insight	Fluctuates; May be present in lucid moments	Absent
Judgment	Poor	Poor May be socially inappropriate
Memory	Impaired	Impaired
Perception	Hallucinations, illusions	No change
Attention	Impaired	Intact — may focus on one thing
Sleep	Disturbed	Normal
Behavior	Agitated Restless	Fluctuates; Agitated, Apathetic Wander

is associated with grieving for losses that combines with other factors to culminate in a full-blown depression. Depression in elderly persons may appear to be or manifest itself as a pseudodementia. Once the depression is treated and lifted, the dementia also should dissipate.

CHARACTERISTICS OF CONFUSION

Because of differences in patients' personality structure and the variety of possible causative factors, each patient's confusion is unique in how it is manifested. Confused patients generally have problems with cognitive functioning, which includes attention span (poor concentration), decision making (impaired judgment), memory (impaired short/long term memory), speech (tangential/illogical content), and thought content (delusions, confabulation).

General Picture of Confusion

The general picture of the patient who is confused may be as follows:

- The patient may have difficulty remembering recent events before or during the hospitalization.

  Patients may not remember what they are being told about their condition or care.

  They may not remember instructions given to them.

In addition, past memory may be affected.

- The patient may deny that any problems exist and confabulate, becoming quite agitated when confronted with their behavior.

  The patient may be disoriented about time, place, and possibly person.

  Patients may misidentify day with night, day of the week, or date of the month and year.

  They may not know where they are; this state may fluctuate–sometimes they are accurate, sometimes not.

  In situations of severe disorientation, patients may not know who they are, although this condition is rare.

  More commonly, patients do not know who you are and need reminding of your name and role at each interaction.

- Disorientation usually becomes more severe as evening comes, a condition referred to as sundowning.

  With decreases in light and stimulation at night, the patient is less able to distinguish between stimuli.

  Increased agitation can be associated with sundowning.

- The patient may have impaired thought processes.
- Patients may show a lack of good judgment, be apathetic, show evidence of illogical thinking, seem deficient in their fund of general knowledge, and be unable to perform simple mathematical calculations.
- The patient may be suspicious, paranoid, scared, frightened, and out of touch with reality.
- The patient's speaking may be affected and sometimes may become strange and bizarre.
- Motor coordination and the ability to walk or lift may be impaired.
- Facial expressions and changes in affect may be inappropriate.
- The patient may be regressed behaviorally, experience loss of control over bodily functions such as bladder or bowel functions, or have a specific body part affected because of brain damage.
- Some patients may be incapable of performing basic activities of daily living and need complete care and monitoring.
- Patients may express themselves inappropriately sexually, perhaps disrobing compulsively or masturbating publicly.

The potential reversibility of some or all of these problems depends on the causative factor. An acute delirium caused by drugs or alcohol should dissipate with time and detoxification. A more chronic problem such as cardiovascular problems or Alzheimer's disease will result in continuous deficits of varying degrees.

RELATED PROBLEMS AND PREDISPOSING FACTORS

Associated problems and predisposing factors of confusion include the following:

- Metabolic, endocrine, and electrolyte disturbances
- Respiratory distress, hypoxia
- Chronic liver and kidney disorders
- Neurologic disorders, epilepsy, Parkinson's disease, and CNS infections (e.g., meningitis, encephalitis, syphilis)
- Cancers, tumors
- Cerebrovascular disease
- Systemic infections (e.g., AIDS)
- Nutritional imbalances, vitamin and mineral poisoning or deficiency
- Injury, trauma, embolism

- Toxic effects: substance abuse, alcohol abuse, adverse reactions to medications
- Sensory overload, sensory deprivation, perceptual problems
- Genetic and birth defects, Down syndrome, Huntington's chorea, multiple sclerosis
- Depression

Elderly Patients

Although confusion has causes and occurs in persons of all ages, its prevalence is higher among elderly patients. Aging is a natural process of change in all body organs and potential functioning that may lead to deficits in cognition. Elderly persons have more potential for disease because illness can manifest itself in later life and because a body that is older and has a diminished capacity is more subject to potential ill health. For whatever reason, elderly patients are at greater risk for confusion.

Elderly patients also frequently have physical changes that increase their susceptibility to the potency or toxic effects of certain medications. Even medications a person has been taking for a long time can pose new problems because of age-related bodily changes. Some confused elderly persons may wander and be a danger for themselves if they are lost. Bone changes may pose another danger of potential injury. Visual and hearing acuity may lessen, posing another potential threat to high-level functioning. The elderly patient may succumb to certain psychiatric disorders, such as depression, due to the losses that are associated with aging.

If confusion is associated with a problem caused by aging, special concerns and care may need to be considered. Do not automatically write off a confused elderly patient as senile and incapable of understanding or improving his communication. He needs to be examined to determine any potentially reversible causes for the confusion.

Alzheimer's Disease

When we think of a chronic dementia in aging or one known to have a presenile onset, Alzheimer's disease comes to mind. Since the mid-1980s, this disease has been highly publicized and as a result is now somewhat better understood.

The disease begins with sporadic losses of memory and forgetfulness, and impairment becomes greater over time. The patient has an impaired ability to learn new information or to recall previously learned information (*DSM-IV-TR*, 2000).

They also have cognitive deficits in the following areas:

- Aphasia-language disturbance
- Apraxia-ability to carry out motor activities despite intact sensory function
- Agnosia-ability to recognize or identify objects despite intact sensory function
- Disturbance in executive functioning-planning, organizing, sequencing, abstracting (DSM-IV-TR, 2000)

Sometimes inappropriate mood fluctuations, perhaps some paranoia, disorientation, speech impairments, and motor impairments all contribute adversely to the person's conscious awareness and cognitive thinking.

Nursing care of patients who have Alzheimer's disease must be concerned with communication patterns and with the effects confusion may have on the patients' safety.

DSM-IV-TR DIAGNOSES

In the past, various different sources from medicine, neurology, psychiatry, and nursing have been inconsistent in their definitions of terms related to confusion, clouded consciousness, and impaired cognition. Many of the discrepancies were based on primary diagnoses, causative factors, or functional descriptions.

DSM-IV-TR lists the following diagnoses relate to confusional states:

- Delirium due to... (indicate the general medical condition)
- Substance intoxication delirium
- Substance withdrawal delirium
- Delirium due to multiple etiologies
- Delirium not otherwise specified
- Dementia of the Alzheimer's type, with early onset:
  Uncomplicated
  With delirium
  With delusions
  With depressed mood
- Dementia of the Alzheimer's type, with late onset:
  Uncomplicated
  With delirium
  With delusions
  With depressed mood
- Vascular dementia:
  Uncomplicated
  With delirium
  With delusions
  With depressed mood
- Dementia due to HIV disease
- Dementia due to head trauma
- Dementia due to Parkinson's disease
- Dementia due to Huntington's disease
- Dementia due to Pick's disease
- Dementia due to Creutzfeldt-Jakob disease
- Dementia due to... (indicate the general medical condition not listed in the preceding)
- Substance-induced persisting dementia
- Dementia due to multiple etiologies
- Dementia not otherwise specified

NANDA NURSING DIAGNOSES

NANDA nursing diagnoses for patients who have confusion may include the following:

- Anxiety
- Impaired memory*
- Risk for injury
- Chronic low self-esteem
- Situational low self-esteem
- Disturbed sensory perception
- Disturbed thought processes
- Risk for other-directed violence
- Risk for self-directed violence

NURSING INTERVENTIONS

Regardless of the precipitant for a patient's confusion, nursing interventions should be implemented from the outset.

The following nursing interventions can be used for patients who are confused:

Intervention: Assess the patient's level of confusion or disorientation by doing a mental status examination.

Rationale: The amount of confusion and its possible cause will help determine the patient's needs and abilities.

Intervention: Offer patients support and provide reassurance.

Rationale: Support and reassurance can increase patients' trust in you and give them a feeling of safety and security.

Intervention: Treat confused patients with dignity and respect.

* most common

- Use their proper names.
- Do not treat them as if they were children.

Rationale: Being treated with dignity and respect increases patients' self-esteem and self-concept.

Intervention: Do reality testing with the patient.

Rationale: Monitoring the fluctuations in the patient's level of awareness and comprehension enables you to make necessary changes in the care plan.

Intervention: Reorient the patient:

- Use calendars, a clock, the newspaper, radio, television, or yourself.
- Make frequent visits.
- Devise memory assistance tools, such as placing the patient's name on his door.

Rationale: Helping patients maintain a reality base can decrease deficits from memory impairment and increase the patients' ability to feel safe and aware.

Intervention: Give positive feedback for correct responses and appropriate independent behaviors.

Rationale: Positive feedback can reinforce appropriate behavior and increase patients' feelings of self-esteem.

Intervention: Provide an environment that keeps the patient safe from injury and potential self-harm.

Rationale: Highest priority. A safe environment decreases the potential for trauma and accidents.

Intervention: Decrease environmental stimuli.

Rationale: Increases in stimuli can increase patients' anxiety, which can compound their inability to comprehend correctly.

Intervention: Use simple communications, simple words, short sentences; be frequently repetitious.

- Large signs for bathroom and room number.
- Big-print calendar.
- Signs in the hallway to the dining room and nursing station.

Rationale: Clear communications can increase patients' ability to comprehend, remember, and follow directions. Helping patients remember and maintain orientation increases their independence.

Intervention: Encourage independence in choices and functioning.

Rationale: Making choices and functioning independently can increase patients' feelings of self-worth and improve their ability to rely on themselves.

Intervention: Administer psychotropic medications as ordered, but judiciously.

Rationale: Decreasing anxiety, psychosis, and depression can relieve patients' confusion or level of confusion and comprehension. Judicious administration is called for because these medications can increase the confusion and add or intensify a delirium. Because of the potential side effects, treatment with some psychopharmacologic agents may be unsuccessful in the elderly patients.

Intervention: Use soft restraints when necessary, but check them often.

Patients must be monitored to avoid injury caused by:

- The restraints themselves,
- By fighting against them, or
- As a result of sequelae of stasis.

Rationale: Restraints may be the last safety measure used for patients who wander and are potentially dangerous to their own health or have a serious and imminent potential for assaultiveness.

Intervention: Provide the patient's family with information on confusion and its underlying causes and treatment.

Rationale: The patient's family may be worried or angry because of the patient's confusion.

CASE STUDY

Mrs. Gold, a 69-year-old woman, was admitted to a medical unit with a diagnosis of pneumonia of the left lung. Mr. Gold, the patient's husband, was out of town on an extended business trip when the couple's daughter-in-law, Joan, noted that Mrs. Gold was quite fatigued, breathless at times, and complaining of chest pain. Joan brought Mrs. Gold to the hospital emergency department because Mrs. Gold did not have a regular physician and apparently had not had a checkup in many years.

Mrs. Gold was admitted to her room at 4:30 p.m., and after a few minutes visiting, Joan left her mother-in-law and went home. Jim was Mrs. Gold's primary nurse for the evening shift, and he went to her room at 5 p.m. to do an initial assessment. Mrs. Gold was not in her room; she was found standing in front of a patient's room two doors down the hallway. Jim escorted Mrs. Gold back to her room and did a nursing assessment.

The assessment included a mini-mental status examination, which Jim thought the patient had a great deal of difficulty answering. He decided to do a more complete mental status examination and was continually concerned with Mrs. Gold's level of confusion. Jim then accurately intervened as follows. He

- *oriented Mrs. Gold to the unit and to her room;*
- *labeled Mrs. Gold's room number with her name;*
- *oriented Mrs. Gold to time, place, and person;*
- *wrote down his own name and the telephone number of Mrs. Gold's daughter-in-law (which he got from the chart) on a piece of paper and taped the paper to Mrs. Gold's bedside stand;*
- *notified the physician of his findings and concerns;*
- *charted the findings of the mental status examination;*
- *alerted the other staff members to Mrs. Gold's confusion problem; and*
- *checked on Mrs. Gold every 15-30 min, assessing her and orienting her as needed.*

The reason for Mrs. Gold's confusion was not immediately apparent or determined. There were no old records to document her mental state. No physician knew her, her husband was out of town, and her daughter-in-law was already in transit. In time, with a thorough workup done for this problem, a cause and perhaps a cure would be found. Nevertheless, in the interim, Mrs. Gold's safety needed to be monitored.

SUMMARY

Despite the precipitant for the confusion, nursing interventions could be implemented from the outset. Nursing personnel need to be knowledgeable about the problem of confusion and the management of confused patients.

EXAM QUESTIONS

CHAPTER 8

Questions 47-50

47. A metabolic disturbance, substance abuse, and trauma are all problems that can precipitate

    a. schizophrenia.
    b. delirium.
    c. dementia.
    d. Alzheimer's disease.

48. The three manifestations of Alzheimer's disease are

    a. impaired ability to learn new information, language disturbance, impaired ability to recognize objects.
    b. loss of memory, loss of sleep, loss of self-esteem.
    c. mood swings, mental illness, anorexia.
    d. loss of memory, mood swings, bulimia.

49. The most common nursing diagnoses related to confusion is

    a. anxiety.
    b. risk for injury.
    c. chronic low self-esteem.
    d. impaired memory.

50. The highest priority in the management of a confused 86-year-old woman is

    a. hygiene.
    b. orientation.
    c. safety.
    d. privacy.

CHAPTER 9

NURSING MANAGEMENT OF THE PATIENT WITH AN EATING DISORDER

CHAPTER OBJECTIVE

After completing this chapter, the reader will be able to recognize the manifestations of the eating disorders anorexia nervosa and bulimia nervosa, and intervene appropriately.

LEARNING OBJECTIVES

After studying this chapter, the reader will be able to

1. discuss the theories of causation for eating disorders.
2. specify signs and symptoms of anorexia nervosa and bulimia nervosa.
3. list NANDA nursing and *DSM-IV-TR* diagnoses that may apply to patients who have eating disorders.
4. recognize treatment options and nursing interventions for eating disorders.

OVERVIEW

Anorexia nervosa and bulimia nervosa are two psychobiological eating disorders that have grown to epidemic proportions. Anorexia nervosa, the oldest, better known of the two disorders, may include self-starvation to the point of emaciation because of a distorted self-image of being fat.

Some evidence in medical history fosters a psychosocial belief that women have attempted for many years to gain some mastery over men or control over their own lives and destinies through self-starvation. In those times when women were suppressed, when they had little or no independence or power, the ability to control one's weight and health may have been seen as a powerful tool. Many of us remember the scene in *Gone with the Wind* in which Scarlett O'Hara and her mammy have a power struggle over what to eat and when. This type of power struggle has been played out for various reasons many times.

Historically, anorexia nervosa was reported only occasionally. However, since the 1970s anorexia nervosa and bulimia nervosa have become almost common problems. In 1985, the third revised edition of the *Diagnostic and Statistical Manual of Mental Disorders* included bulimia nervosa as a separate disease with its own definitions and treatment considerations. The binge-purge cycle previously considered part of the syndrome of anorexia nervosa now is seen regularly in young women on college campuses. Some think anorexia nervosa and bulimia nervosa are two parts of a continuous disease process that have some similar and some different signs and symptoms. The severity and danger of these signs and symptoms vary from person to person.

Society contributes to the occurrence of these disorders by fostering a goal of what young women ought to look like. Currently it is popular to be thin as well as body conscious. This socialization and acceptance of a norm have helped hide the dangers of these diseases.

Patients who have anorexia nervosa may be seen on general hospital units when they have become so thin that their lives may be in jeopardy, and medical interventions along with, or independent of, psychiatric treatment are necessary to sustain life. Patients who have bulimia nervosa generally maintain their weight at a level that is close to average or slightly less than normal weight. Generally the risk of death is minimal.

PREVALENCE

It is estimated that the lifetime prevalence of anorexia nervosa is 0.5% of the female population. Among males, the incidence is approximately one-tenth that among females. Bulimia nervosa, which is more common than anorexia, is estimated to occur in 1-3% of the female population. In males, it is approximately one-tenth of the occurrence in females. The age of onset of these eating disorders is during adolescence or early adult life. The incidence of both has increased in recent decades (*DSM-IV-TR*, 2000).

THEORIES OF CAUSATION

The eating disorders have no known causes, despite commonalties from patient to patient. Some acknowledged beliefs for causative factors exist, and, as in other areas of psychiatry, research in this area is ongoing.

There is a genetic or familial pattern for eating disorders. There is a greater risk among first-degree biological relatives with eating disorders than among the general population (*DSM-IV-TR*, 2000).

Physiologic theories include the possibility of neuroendocrine and neurotransmitter abnormalities, particularly an increase in serotonin activity. For example, studies have indicated that bulimics have low serotonin levels that may predispose them to binge-eating cycles.

Developmental theory proposes a developmental crisis as the cause. Perhaps some block or stoppage in a child's developmental level during the oral stage of growth leaves the child dependent, unable to separate appropriately and unable to succeed. Adolescence may be another stage for a possible developmental crisis. Because so many patients with anorexia nervosa begin to have signs and symptoms during their early teens, it seems possible that the disease is a pathologic development of an adolescent in turmoil. Self-concept, identity, and body image are so important during adolescence.

A possible psychological cause or interpretation of self-starvation is that the self-gratification and pleasure attached to eating are equated with selfishness and evil. Controlling the natural drive to eat symbolically represents the struggle of the will over more basic needs and desires.

Anorexia nervosa can also represent a rejection of one's own sexuality or be a punishment for real or imagined transgressions. Nearly starving oneself to death can be a severe denial of the self and the right to exist.

Sociologic theories look at the control factor. Perhaps anorexia nervosa is an attempt to exert control over parents. Family treatment often is included as part of a total treatment regimen. The environmental influence of the media on thinness may be a factor. In some cultures, ours being one, thinness is highly desired and is a contributing factor.

Most likely, a combination of events determines what causes eating disorders and to what extent they are manifested.

TABLE 9-1: ESSENTIAL FEATURES OF ANOREXIA NERVOSA AND BULIMIA NERVOSA	
Anorexia Nervosa	**Bulimia Nervosa**
Refusal to maintain body weight at or above a minimally normal weight for age and height (e.g., weight loss leading to maintenance of body weight less than 85% of that expected; or Failure to make expected weight gain during period of growth, leading to body weight less than 85% of that expected).	Recurrent episodes of binge eating. An episode of binge eating is characterized by both of the following: 1. Eating, in a discrete period of time (e.g., within any 2-hour period), an amount of food that is definitely larger than most people would eat during a similar period of time and under similar circumstances 2. A sense of lack of control over eating during the episode (e.g., a feeling that one cannot stop eating or control what or how much one is eating)
Intense fear of gaining weight or becoming fat, even though underweight.	Recurrent inappropriate compensatory behavior in order to prevent weight gain, such as: • Self-induced vomiting; • Misuse of laxatives, • Diuretics, enemas, or other medications; fasting; or • Excessive exercise.
Disturbance in the way in which: • One's body weight or shape is experienced, • Undue influence of body weight or shape on self-evaluation, • Denial of the seriousness of the current low body weight.	The binge eating and inappropriate compensatory behaviors both occur, on average, at least twice a week for 3 months.
In post-menarcheal females, amenorrhea, i.e., the absence of at least three consecutive menstrual cycles. (A woman is considered to have amenorrhea if her periods occur only following hormone, e.g., estrogen administration.)	Self-evaluation is unduly influenced by body shape and weight.
	The disturbance does not occur exclusively during episodes of anorexia nervosa.

Note. Eating Disorders. Diagnostic and Statistical Manual of Mental Disorders, Fourth Edition, Text Revision, by the American Psychiatric Association. 2000, Washington, DC: American Psychiatric Association. Adapted with permission.

SIGNS AND SYMPTOMS

Anorexia Nervosa

Although anorexia and bulimia nervosa have many signs and symptoms, with some overlap and some differences in intensity, the following criteria are generally included as necessary for the diagnosis of anorexia nervosa (refer to Table 9-1):

- A disturbance in body image
- An intense fear of gaining weight that is not relieved after weight loss occurs
- A body weight of 85% or less of the expected norm
- An absence of menses in postmenarcheal females (*DSM-IV-TR*, 2000).

The disorder manifests itself in the following ways:

- A refusal to eat anything or anything of substance
- A severe weight loss with emaciation often described as a waiflike appearance or looking like a "concentration camp victim"
- A preoccupation with food, reading food magazines, cooking elaborate meals for others but not eating any of the food prepared
- Strange and bizarre food habits, (e.g., stealing and hoarding food, though not eating it, or setting places at the table in a specific and compulsive manner)
- Hyperactivity and excessive exercising
- Abuse of diuretics and laxatives
- Chronic constipation
- Skin changes: a yellow tinge or the appearance of lanugo, a fine downy hair; hyperkeratosis
- Loss of hair or changes in its texture (e.g., brittle and dry)
- Hypothermia and bradycardia
- Hypotension
- Leukopenia
- Anemia
- Hypoglycemia
- Hypoproteinemia
- Increased basal metabolic rate
- Malnutrition
- Dehydration
- Electrolyte disturbances
- Abnormal thyroid function
- Abnormal adrenal cortical function (*DSM-IV-TR*, 2000).

Emotionally, patients who are anorexic often are depressed and anxious. Sometimes they are psychotic, and sometimes they have obsessive-compulsive traits. Some have committed suicide, and all anorexic patients should be evaluated for this potential.

If a person dies from being anorexic, it is generally a person who is chronically ill and dies from starvation or committing suicide.

Bulimia Nervosa

A person who has bulimia nervosa gorges on food repetitively and uncontrollably in a short time; this is the binge. Caloric intake during a binge is high. Foods usually favored are high in sugar and fat. The binge ends with purging or self-induced vomiting, usually accomplished by sticking a finger down one's throat.

When this is done repetitively, over a long time, a reflexive, uncontrollable pattern of vomiting may develop. In addition to purging by self-induced vomiting, the person may use and abuse diuretics and/or laxatives, diet pills and steroids, and excessive exercise.

Although the binge-purge cycle is the key element in bulimia nervosa, other characteristic signs and symptoms include the following (refer to Table 9-1):

- Chronic dieting with weight fluctuations
- A problem with body image, usually with distortion and some obsessive concerns
- Stomachaches, potential ulcers, and other chronic gastrointestinal disorders
- Frequent sore throats
- Dental problems (with extensive purging, the calcium of the teeth is worn away by the stomach acid)
- Rectal bleeding
- Malnutrition, electrolyte imbalances, and vitamin deficiencies (*DSM-IV-TR*, 2000).

Characteristics of ending the binge include the following:

- Falling asleep
- Being caught while purging
- Being found hiding and gorging

- Having stomachaches and stomach pains

If a person dies from bulimia nervosa, it is usually from hypokalemia or suicide. There is a less favorable prognosis for patients who are bulimic than anorexic.

DSM-IV-TR DIAGNOSES

These psychiatric diagnoses may be related to eating disorders:

- Anorexia nervosa
- Bulimia nervosa
- Binge eating disorder

Additional *DSM-IV-TR* diagnoses that may be present:

- Major depressive disorder
- Substance use abuse
- Obsessive-compulsive disorder
- Borderline personality disorder

NANDA NURSING DIAGNOSES

Nursing diagnoses that may be considered for patients with eating disorders include the following:

- Anxiety
- Disturbed body image
- Ineffective coping
- Ineffective denial
- Fatigue
- Deficient fluid volume
- Ineffective health maintenance
- Imbalanced nutrition: less than body requirements
- Powerlessness
- Disturbed thought processes
- Chronic low self-esteem
- Situational low self-esteem
- Risk for self-mutilation
- Social isolation

TREATMENT OPTIONS

Treatment options for the eating disorders differ according to the severity of the illness and the potential danger from adverse sequelae for which the patient is at risk. Treatment is more successful in patients who begin as soon as the eating disorder becomes apparent. Depending on the level of care needed when the patient seeks treatment, many therapists are available on an inpatient or an outpatient basis. Both types of therapy may be necessary, and one or more inpatient stays may be needed during a long course of illness.

For a severely disturbed patient, one who is critically ill because of starvation, medical intervention may be needed first. This may include hospitalization and forced feedings in emergency medical situations.

Long-term treatment for patients with eating disorders is psychiatric therapy. Although no one type of therapy seems particularly more successful, a combination of therapies for a relatively long time, years perhaps, seems to be somewhat successful. Therapies that may be included in the treatment regimen include the following:

- Individual psychotherapy
- Group therapy
- Family therapy
- Behavior modification
- Cognitive therapy
- Relaxation techniques
- Hypnosis
- Education

- Occupational therapy
- Recreational therapy
- Nutritional counseling

Psychopharmacologic therapy generally is not thought to be the best treatment method. Anxiolytics (antianxiety) drugs may be ordered before meals, to help patients with eating. Prokinetic agents may be given to assist with digestion in patients who have delayed gastric emptying. Vitamin supplements may be given adjunctively. If patients have comorbid conditions, such as anxiety or depression, they may be treated with medications for those conditions.

Several eating disorder programs are available. These generally offer inpatient stays as well as outpatient follow-up treatment. Some clinics or residences are attached to hospitals and others are free-standing institutions. Many programs are connected to a wide variety of services and treatment for other problems, such as chemical dependency. Some programs are exclusively for eating disorders.

In a general hospital on a medical unit, nurses may be caring for patients with eating disorders in the capacity of administering basic and supplemental nutrition. The preferred method is for the patient to eat a balanced and nutritionally complete diet. The nurse can confer with the dietitian who will be in charge of this regimen. Additionally, a feeding tube may be necessary to provide supplements to regular meals. The nursing staff generally administers these feedings.

Patients, particularly those who already have a distorted body image, dislike being fed through a tube. Some may try to pull it out, may fight against it, or may have behavioral problems during feeding administrations. The nurse can help by being supportive and reassuring and clarifying that the feedings are required for life support and they are not a punishment.

Patients who are critically ill and in need of great amounts of nutrients or whose gastrointestinal systems cannot tolerate a regular diet or tube feedings may need parenteral nutrition administered through a large vein, such as the subclavian vein. Some patients who need long-term parenteral therapy may have a catheter such as a Hickman catheter implanted surgically into the right atrium. These forms of nutritional support, which may seem extreme, generally are used only in severe situations.

NURSING INTERVENTIONS

The following nursing interventions can be used with a patient who has an eating disorder:

- **Intervention:** Establish a therapeutic relationship and a positive rapport with the patient.

  Rationale: The patient can benefit from the nurse's use of self as a therapeutic tool.
- **Intervention:** Assess the patient's mental status.

  Rationale: The patient's mental status gives a baseline reference and helps in monitoring potential behavioral changes.
- **Intervention:** Assess the patient's nutritional status, intake and output, and weight.

  Rationale: In patients with an eating disorder, reaching and maintaining an optimal level of health and well-being may be determined by the patients' nutritional status.
- **Intervention:** Observe vital signs, especially in patients who may be at critically low weights.

  Rationale: Eating disorders can be fatal diseases.
- **Intervention:** Observe for suicidal ideation.

  Rationale: Patients who have eating disorders, particularly anorexia nervosa, may become suicidal.
- **Intervention:** Provide one-to-one supervision during meals.
  - Observe the patient closely for any indication of hiding food.

- Give the patient 30 min to eat.
- Do not encourage the patient to eat during this time.

Rationale: Patients with an eating disorder are ambivalent about food. They may take a long time to eat and may attempt to hide food to avoid eating or to gorge with later.

- **Intervention:** Encourage the patient to approach a health care team member if they feel the need to purge.

  Rationale: Expressions of feelings can help reduce the patient's anxiety, and identify alternatives to vomiting.

- **Intervention:** Administer supplemental feedings and medications as ordered.

  Rationale: Supplemental feedings and medication help the patient achieve a satisfactory nutritional status.

- **Intervention:** Provide support and reassurance.

  Rationale: Patients may feel out of control.

- **Intervention:** Encourage patients to verbalize their feelings.

  Rationale: Verbalization of feelings can reduce stress and clarify problems.

- **Intervention:** Allow ventilation of feelings of anger.

  Rationale: Some patients experience a great deal of anger and suppress it; this anger needs to be released in an appropriate manner.

- **Intervention:** Observe for potential sabotage of the treatment plan.

  Rationale: Fears of gaining weight and the existence of long-standing habits may cause some patients to sabotage their treatment. Patients with eating disorders may induce vomiting, use laxatives, and throw away food while hospitalized.

- **Intervention:** Observe for signs and symptoms of anxiety, depression, and psychosis.

  Rationale: Anxiety, depression, and psychosis may be present in patients who have eating disorders.

- **Intervention:** Collaborate with other health care providers, such as physicians, social service workers, and dietitians.

  Rationale: Collaboration with other health care providers is necessary to establish and use a working treatment plan.

CASE STUDY

A 20-year-old woman was admitted to a medical unit of a general hospital for treatment of malnutrition. She weighed 74 lb (33.6 kg) and was 5 ft (1.5 m) tall. She denied being anorexic and claimed to have a problem of low energy — "a definite no-no for an aspiring ballerina," she would say.

The patient's primary nurse correctly believed that the patient had anorexia nervosa and was denying the problem. When the primary nurse discussed her concerns with the patient's physician, he confirmed her suspicions, adding, "I recommended psychiatric consultation, but she refused. She would only agree to come to the hospital for a 'rest and overhaul,' as she put it. I was concerned about her and thought she should come in anyway."

The hospital had a clinical nurse specialist in psychiatric and mental health nursing on the staff with whom the primary nurse previously had collaborated. She called her and discussed the nursing care for this patient. A nursing staff meeting was scheduled for a few days later. In the meanwhile, the psychiatric nursing specialist visited the patient and remained in contact with the primary nurse.

Later in the week, at the nursing conference, the following information was shared:

The patient appeared much younger than her stated age of 20. She had long, straight, brown hair, which lacked luster and was stringy and sparse. She appeared waiflike, with wide eyes and a hollow, gaunt face. Her affect was sad. She appeared anxious and paced around the unit, dragging a portable IV pole behind her. The pole carried a bag with a catheter connected to a nasogastric feeding tube.

The nurses who knew the patient agreed that she seemed "strange." She talked incessantly about food but barely ate anything. She was highly aware of the nasogastric tube, and at meal times, she was withdrawn and preoccupied. Sometimes she would have her eyes closed and she would be muttering. The primary nurse thought that the patient was hallucinating at times, because she had noticed the patient gesturing and muttering in a peculiar manner. She was concerned with the patient's denial of the eating disorder.

The patient had many of the distressing signs and symptoms of anorexia nervosa. Her behavior was cause for concern. She had been seen taking laxatives surreptitiously, throwing some food away from her regular meal tray, attempting to exercise by doing sit-ups and push-ups, and even attempting a cartwheel when she was temporarily free of tubes and monitors. Additionally, some of the nursing staff thought they had heard her vomiting in the bathroom.

A general medical unit usually is not prepared to provide the wide range of therapeutic options for a patient who has an eating disorder. It was recommended at the nursing conference that the following occur:

- The clinical nurse specialist confers with the patient's primary physician about obtaining a psychiatric evaluation.
- The primary nurse establishes a positive therapeutic relationship with the patient and discusses the signs and symptoms of the patient's illness with her.

In addition, the primary nurse could educate the patient about anorexia nervosa and set mutually agreeable goals for this hospitalization.

The general nursing staff should:

- observe the patient's behavior and mood;
- evaluate her via a mental status examination;
- measure the patient's intake and output and weigh her daily;
- observe the patient during mealtimes without encouraging her to eat. Give her 30 min to eat and then remove the tray;
- administer feedings via a nasogastric tube as ordered;
- maintain open channels of communication; include the patient, her physician, her family, the clinical nurse specialist, and the dietitian;
- document the patient's mental status, medical status, nutritional requirements, vital signs, and intake and output;
- document all interventions carefully and clearly; and
- be consistent in their approach when following the patient's care plan.

The staff will need to continually evaluate the effectiveness of their care plan.

SUMMARY

Anorexia nervosa is characterized by a refusal to maintain body weight at or above a minimally normal weight for age and height, or failure to make expected weight gain during a period of normal growth. Bulimia nervosa is characterized by episodes of binge eating, a sense of a lack of control, use of recurrent inappropriate compensatory behavior in order to prevent weight gain, and over concern with body shape. Patients who experience these disorders suffer from a variety of physiologic problems that may cause death. The nursing care will differ from patient to patient depending upon the severity of the illnesses.

EXAM QUESTIONS

CHAPTER 9

Questions 51-56

51. An adolescent developmental crisis is a theoretical cause for
    a. anorexia nervosa.
    b. schizophrenia.
    c. schizoaffective disorder.
    d. personality disorder.

52. The key element in bulimia nervosa is
    a. malnutrition.
    b. psychosis.
    c. binge-purge cycle.
    d. weight loss.

53. Signs and symptoms of anorexia nervosa are
    a. a physical illness, fear of obesity, and a weight loss of 25 lb (11.4 kg).
    b. a weight loss of 25 lb and galactorrhea.
    c. intense fear of obesity and a weight gain of 25 lb.
    d. disturbance in body image and an intense fear of gaining weight.

54. The signs and symptoms of bulimia nervosa are
    a. binging-purging and skin changes.
    b. headaches and dehydration.
    c. dry, brittle hair; self-induced vomiting.
    d. stomachaches, binging-purging.

55. The nursing diagnosis, disturbed body image, would be indicative of
    a. organic brain disorder.
    b. anxiety disorder.
    c. personality disorder.
    d. eating disorder.

56. A combination of therapies, such as individual and group therapy, behavior modification, and nutritional counseling, are appropriate treatments for
    a. schizoaffective disorder.
    b. obsessive-compulsive disorder.
    c. anorexia nervosa.
    d. bipolar-affective disorder.

CHAPTER 10

NURSING MANAGEMENT OF THE POTENTIALLY AGGRESSIVE PATIENT

CHAPTER OBJECTIVE

After completing this chapter, the reader will be able to recognize patients who are potentially aggressive and apply nursing interventions that can be used to prevent workplace violence.

LEARNING OBJECTIVES

After studying this chapter, the reader will be able to

1. know the factors that increase the potential for workplace violence.
2. recognize the early warning signs of workplace violence involving an aggressive patient.
3. describe the purpose of chemical and mechanical restraints and the procedures for using them with aggressive patients.
4. list the NANDA nursing diagnoses and *DSM-IV-TR* disorders that often are present in aggressive patients.
5. specify the nursing responsibilities related to managing patients who are assaultive or have the potential for engaging in workplace violence.

OVERVIEW

Rage, anger, and hostility are powerful and sometimes frightening emotions to have, as well as to confront in patients. The potential violence that may erupt because of these emotions can be quite scary for nursing personnel. Psychiatric nursing personnel are trained in the management of aggressive behavior and crises involving escalation. Usually, nurses in a general hospital are not; often members of the security staff in acute care settings manage the occasional escalation of an aggressive patient.

The Occupational Safety and Health Act of 1970 requires that each employer shall furnish to each of his employees employment and a place of employment which are free from recognized hazards that are causing or are likely to cause death or serious physical harm to his employees (OSH, 2003). This requires health care institutions to take the necessary precautions to protect nursing personnel from workplace violence.

FACTORS THAT MAY INCREASE THE RISK OF WORKPLACE VIOLENCE

Workplace violence ranges from offensive or threatening language to homicide. Incidents of violence are episodes or outbursts that involve hitting, choking, or generally assaulting another person; damaging property; throwing cups; smashing IV bottles; and so forth. One of the difficulties with providing a safe environment is that sickness and potential life-threatening factors cause stress in patients, their family members, and personnel in health care workplaces. Such stress can aggravate factors that lead to violence; the levels of which are reportedly on the increase in society in general, and in health care workplaces in particular.

Research demonstrates that among health care personnel, nursing staff are most at risk of workplace violence. The risk factors for violence vary with each health care facility depending on location, size, and type of care. Common risk factors for workplace violence are listed in Table 10-1.

Workplace violence is destructive and has a profoundly negative impact upon nurses. Nurses may suffer physical injuries, psychological trauma, such as anger, depression, fear, self-blame, and powerlessness, and increased stress and anxiety, or death. This can affect the institution by causing loss of job satisfaction, low worker morale, increased job stress and increased staff turnover rate (NIOSH, 2002).

Members of the nursing staff should have some guidelines for dealing with aggression, just as they do for a fire or other disaster's. These guidelines should be based on a team approach with the security staff, because both security and nursing staff members are present and needed in these situations. Nursing home personnel, because of both the frequency of incidents and the delicate nature of some patients' conditions, should have training in the management of potentially aggressive patients.

Incidents

Recent data indicate that hospital workers are at high risk for experiencing violence in the workplace. The National Institute for Occupational Safety and Health (NIOSH, 2002, http://www.cdc.gov/niosh/2002-101.html) reported that nonfatal assaults on hospital workers were at a rate of 8.3 assaults per 10,000 workers. This rate is much higher than the rate of nonfatal assaults for all private-sector industries, which are 2 per 10,000 workers.

DSM-IV-TR DIAGNOSES

Patients considered more at risk for becoming aggressive are those who have had a violent outburst before. Aggressive patients most often have the following *DSM-IV-TR* mental disorders:

- Organic brain syndromes/organic mental syndromes
- Alzheimer's disease
- Multi-infarct dementia
- Alcohol and other drug use, abuse, or withdrawal
- Substance abuse disorders
- Schizophrenia
- Borderline personality disorder

NANDA NURSING DIAGNOSES

The nursing diagnoses that are often considered with patients who are potentially violent are as follows:

- Impaired verbal communication
- Acute confusion
- Chronic confusion
- Defensive coping
- Ineffective coping
- Impaired environmental interpretation
- Fear
- Hopelessness
- Impaired memory
- Noncompliance
- Powerlessness
- Chronic low self-esteem

TABLE 10-1: FACTORS THAT MAY INCREASE THE RISK OF WORK-RELATED VIOLENCE

Patients and Visitors	Staff	Environment
Acutely disturbed, violent or volatile patients	Lack of training in recognition and management of escalating, hostile and assaultive behavior, or potentially volatile patients	Poor or inadequate security measures
Patients with a history of violence or certain psychotic diagnoses	Low staffing levels during times of specific increased activity such as meal times, visiting hours, and change of shift	Poorly lit corridors, rooms, parking lots, and other areas
Patients who are on criminal holds by police and the criminal justice system	Solo work, particularly in remote locations	Highly accessible worksites with little or no privacy
Trauma patients	Interventions demanding close physical contact such as examinations, treatments or transporting patients	Unrestricted movement of the public in clinics and hospitals
Drug or alcohol abusers or patients under the influence	Shift work, including commuting to and from work at night	Long waits in emergency or clinic areas which are overcrowded and uncomfortable
Distraught family members	Demanding workloads	The availability of drugs or money at hospitals, clinics, and pharmacies, making them likely robbery targets
Presence of gang members	The use of temporary and inexperienced staff; Working alone	The prevalence of handguns and other weapons Home visiting with its associated isolation

Note. National Institute for Occupational Safety and Health (NIOSH). (2002). *VIOLENCE Occupational Hazards in Hospitals DHHS* (Publication No. 2002–101) by the National Institute of Occupational Safety and Health (NIOSH). (2002). From: http://www.cdc.gov/niosh/2002-101.html

- Situational low self-esteem
- Self-mutilation
- Risk for self-mutilation
- Disturbed sensory perception
- Impaired social interaction
- Risk for suicide
- Disturbed thought processes
- Risk for other-directed violence
- Risk for self-directed violence

ASSESSMENT

Nurse's Self-Awareness

You need to be aware of how you deal with angry patient's. For example, if you become angry yourself, you will not be therapeutic and you will be unable to defuse a patient's aggression. Instead, you will more likely intensify the patient's emotions. If you are over controlling, you may get into a power struggle with the patient. If you withdraw from an angry patient, you will be ineffective. If the patient is escalating angry feelings, he is communicating to you that he is losing control, and needs help regaining impulse control.

Never overlook your own feelings of anxiety during a conversation or confrontation with a patient. If your intuition tells you that this patient may become dangerous or that the situation may be getting out of hand and potentially beyond your control, do the following:

- SEEK HELP EARLY.
- Consider yourself a good monitor of a potential crisis.
- Pay attention to your gut reactions.
- Anticipate potential problems.
- Know your patients' history as well as their current problems.
- Be alert to patients whose primary or secondary diagnoses are associated with a high degree of potential for violent occurrences.

EARLY WARNING SIGNS

You need to consider the source and target of the patient's anger, and the likelihood of escalation. Potentially violent patients often are demanding, argumentative, hostile, and perhaps challenging and blatantly threatening. This behavior may be directed toward staff members, other patients, or the patients' family and friends, depending on the situation. A person seemingly in authority is often the recipient of this type of verbal abuse, although anyone who is in the way may be the target of a patient who cannot control himself or herself.

Patients who are potentially violent may exhibit the following behaviors:

- Become extremely loud; start shouting.
- Become physically tense; appear rigid and tight.
- Clench their teeth and hands.
- Be quite agitated, seemingly anxious and restless; perhaps pacing if mobile; seeming quite jittery.
- Have a labile mood, but exhibit mostly anger.

PRELIMINARY ACTIONS

The nursing staff should manage patients who are testy and seem to have the potential for violence carefully. The following steps are important to remember in these situations:

- Maintain your behavior in a way that helps diffuse anger. Present a calm, caring attitude.
- Give irritable patients choices and options.
- Do not be demanding and argumentative; perhaps some rules or procedures can be waived temporarily. Patients who are angry and potentially violent generally feel helpless and powerless. They need help with their self-control.
- To avoid power struggles with these patients do not confront them. This approach will help deescalate the patients' behavior and the situation.
- Open and consistent communication should be ongoing between staff members and between the patient and the staff. Talk to the patient. Try to find out what is precipitating this crisis.
- Don't match the threats. Don't give orders. Acknowledge the person's feelings (for example, "I know you are frustrated"). Ask what the patient would like done. How can the staff help? How can you, the nurse, help?
- Decrease the stimuli for the patient. The loud and unfamiliar noises of the hospital may be particularly stressful, or bright lights may be bothersome.
- Avoid any behavior that may be interpreted as aggressive (for example, moving rapidly, getting too close, touching, or speaking loudly). Physical touch can be a trigger. Patients may misinterpret the contact and feel threatened with bodily harm, which they may need to defend themselves against. Delay procedures

that may escalate a patient's potentially violent behavior.

- Before the situation gets out of control, check the environment. Look for potentially dangerous objects and remove them if possible. Items such as glasses, scissors, food utensils, and other breakable or sharp objects can be used as weapons.
- Never allow yourself to be alone and vulnerable with a potentially violent patient or trapped in a room away from the exit. Team up with another member of the staff when you see such a patient; there can be safety in numbers.
- Alert other members of the nursing staff of a potential problem. Do not call on new and inexperienced staff members. Additional personnel should be available to help with a crisis.

WHEN VIOLENCE ERUPTS

If the potential for violence escalates, and a patient is behaving in a threatening manner, the nursing staff must take action quickly.

Always seek assistance in an emergency. Get help from the security staff, other nursing personnel, or any other hospital personnel who are available. A patient who has a weapon should be disarmed by persons who are trained to do so. If the patient cannot be disarmed easily, your safety and that of others in the area must be considered. Although you may be able to protect yourself with shields and barriers against knives, this may not be the case if a patient has a loaded gun.

The patient may need to be chemically restrained with prn antianxiety or antipsychotic medication, or physically restrained, or possibly both.

Chemical Restraint

Use of antianxiety or antipsychotic medications is one way of managing a patient's violent episode. The medications most often used are the low-dose, high-potency antipsychotics such as haloperidol (Haldol®) or fluphenazine (Prolixin®) or the short-acting benzodiazepine, lorazepam (Ativan®) or alprazolam (Xanax®). Oral medications may be offered first, but if escalation is rapid, an intramuscular (IM) medication may be necessary.

In some situations, patients may become violent as a result of psychosis and thereby need an antipsychotic. It the patients are also a danger to themselves or others, their agitation will also need to be controlled. Such patients therefore are given both an antipsychotic and antianxiety medications.

Each health care institution has, or should have, some guidelines for the use of medications in potentially violent situations, and all nurses should be aware of this procedure. The medication orders may read as follows:

- Haldol 10 mg IM every hr until sedated and/or Ativan 2 mg IM for agitation.

The antipsychotic medication is given as an initial dose, and the patient is observed at 15-min intervals. In some instances, medication may be given as often as every half hour until the violent episode is in check. The patient may be quite willing to take the medication orally. The action of these drugs is slower, however, when they are taken orally. If the situation is moderate, the patient can be offered this alternative route.

Nursing Responsibilities

The nursing responsibilities involved in handling a violent episode by medicating a patient with a potent pharmacologic agent include the following:

- Checking for or obtaining a physician's order to administer this medication.
- Preparing the medication: capsules, tablets, or liquid; IM injection, or IV drip, or butterfly infusion.

- Assessing the patient's vital signs (e.g., blood pressure, pulse, and respiration) before giving the drugs.
- Informing the patient of the procedure to follow and providing reassurance and support if needed.
- After the medication has been administered, observing the patient, assessing for a decrease in signs and symptoms of aggression, and noting any untoward side effects of medication given.
- Periodically checking the patient's vital signs.
- Documenting the incident and the medications given by recording the information in the patient's chart or as the institution directs.

Mechanical Restraint

Sometimes patients need both medications and mechanical restraints to prevent them from harming themselves, or from leaving the hospital precipitously when leaving may be a significant threat to their health. As with protocols for using chemical restraint, each health care institution should have a procedure to follow for physically restraining a patient.

In psychiatric facilities, patients who are restrained mechanically usually are placed in seclusion. Special rooms are set aside for just such an emergency. These rooms generally have no furniture except, perhaps, a mattress or bed and often are soundproof. They can be locked from the outside. A small window in the door allows staff members to check on the patient's safety and well-being. These rooms are stripped of all possible objects that could be used to cause harm to the patient (self-harm) or to others. They provide a quiet place for patients to regain some self-control; all stimuli are decreased.

General hospitals usually do not have such rooms available. Large hospitals with busy emergency departments may have a holding room designated for psychiatry that can be used for this type of seclusion.

When a patient is restrained mechanically in a general hospital, the number of staff members needed and the type of restraint required depend on the patient's size and strength and potential for violence. The general recommendation is that five to six trained staff members are necessary for the hands-on management of a violent patient, in other words, one staff member available to hold each extremity and an additional staff member available to apply the restraints.

Restraint Procedure

The patient is held by his or her arms and legs and walked, carried, or placed in as comfortable a position as possible, usually in a hospital bed with side rails up, and placed in wrist and ankle restraints. These restraints may be cotton, gauze, cloth, or leather, depending on the patient's size and strength.

Ideally, one person should be in charge of a group of five or six staff members. If no one person is in charge, the possibility of mixing up messages with everyone going in different directions, or having different ideas of what needs to be done and how to do it, can produce a disjointed effort. Consequently, the patient may escape and be harmed or do harm. The confusion that ensues when no one is in charge invariably adds to the patient's sense of being out of control and thus escalates the situation.

The best approach toward the patient is a uniform one. All staff members should move or walk toward the patient together. Sometimes this simple show of force and the sheer numbers, subdues a patient. Before the approach is begun, to avoid confusion, the team leader should assign which staff member will hold which extremity.

For maximal control, hold patients firmly just above or below their joints (elbows and knees) when walking them. Use the most secure hold you can. If you need to loosen a patient's grip on you, first try to tug the patient's thumb away gently; the rest of the hand will follow. The staff member or members who may be near the patient's head must be aware that the patient may try to bite them. Be alert.

Staff members should try to be calm themselves. Do not speak loudly; instead be firm and speak slowly, clearly, and precisely. A soft voice may have a quieting effect on the patient.

Whenever mechanical restraint is necessary, be firm.

- Do not negotiate with the patient.
- Do not confuse the patient with too many options.
- Remember, this patient is out of control.
- You may want to say something similar to the following:

  "We feel you are not in good control of yourself right now. We will help you calm down. You need to remain in this bed, and then we can talk."

Remember to check the room for potentially dangerous objects. Remove any watches, glasses, jewelry, shoes, and so forth that could be a hazard. Keep in mind that no place is absolutely free of danger. Patients have broken light bulbs and cut themselves with the shards. One patient used the cord in his pajama waist to hang himself. Be cautious and aware. Look around the area from the patient's eye level so you can see what the patient sees.

If the optimal number of staff members needed to subdue someone safely is not available, or if you are alone in a precarious situation, you may need to use a device as a blockade. You can use a blanket, a sheet, or even a mattress to take someone down to the floor initially or to protect yourself. This maneuver can buy you time or stun the patient temporarily until others arrive to help you apply restraints as needed. REMEMBER: For any of these techniques, training is essential to keep both you and the patient safe.

The safety of the patient and your own safety should be considered at all times. Try to present yourself as not being punitive but as attempting to help the patient regain some self-control over violent behavior.

Patients should be shown respect and allowed to maintain their dignity. Make sure everyone knows the patient's name and uses it. Avoid nicknames or expressions such as the following:

- "Shut up, Mac!"
- "Calm down now, fella."
- "Take it easy, grandpa."

NURSING INTERVENTIONS

The role of the nurse in the management of an aggressive patient will be found within the protocol, policy, or procedure manual of each institution. Within this framework, the following nursing interventions may apply:

- Use good interpersonal skills. Establish a rapport.
- Assess for the potentially violent occurrence.
- Acknowledge the patient's feelings (e.g., You seem angry.)
- Anticipate a potential problem. Trust your judgment.
- If a patient is escalating, communicate verbally with him in a soft but firm voice. Attempt to foster a therapeutic relationship by conveying empathy by acknowledging the patient's feelings.
- Encourage patients to express anger verbally rather than by "acting out" their feelings.
- Be respectful of a patient's personal space.

- Use stress reduction techniques (e.g., deep breathing).
- Continually observe patients who are potentially dangerous to themselves or others.
- Assess the patient's coping skills and ability. Crisis intervention techniques may work early to prevent violent eruption.
- Help the patient maintain control by offering choices, talking, or walking.
- Initiate or collaborate on a plan that includes a team approach to restraining a patient.
- Alert others of the potential problem. Do not approach an aggressive patient alone.
- Monitor the situation for the safety of others and of yourself.
- Follow the individual institution's protocol, policy, or procedure for restraining a patient either mechanically or chemically.
- Document the violent incident and report it to all pertinent members of the health care team.
- After the patient has been restrained, plan future interventions by having a follow-up team meeting or debriefing session to discuss the effectiveness of the restraint procedure. Was it smooth, safe, and effective, or were there many glitches, such as patients not responding positively, or staff members hurt?
- Revise and review the protocol.
- In some states the law requires a legal hold if the patient is restrained with more than a Posey belt or soft restraints. In addition, restraints may necessitate one-on-one observation by staff. It is important to know your hospital's policy and what your state law requires.

CASE STUDY

A 58-year-old man, Mr. Anno, was admitted to a urologic unit for a transurethral resection for his benign prostatic hypertrophy. During the admission intake, Mr. Anno's daughter mentioned his mood swings. Mr. Anno spoke in broken English; Spanish was his native language.

The evening before his surgery, Mr. Anno spoke in an animated manner, in Spanish, to another patient. Twice the evening nurse came to Mr. Anno's bedside to calm him down and see what was wrong. He was gesturing and muttering to himself, quite loudly at times. The physician on call was notified. When the physician examined Mr. Anno, the patient was still animated but not as wild. The physician ordered a sedative, and said he would check again in an hour. Mr. Anno fell asleep in a short while. The rest of the evening shift was unremarkable.

Mr. Anno awoke about 6 a.m. and was given his preoperative medications. He was taken for surgery at 7 a.m. The surgery went well, with no complications. Mr. Anno had an unremarkable recovery, medically, and was returned to his unit at 2 p.m.

Although he appeared somewhat sleepy, Mr. Anno was mumbling to himself and gesturing with his hands. The primary nurse became somewhat concerned when these behaviors seemed to increase and Mr. Anno's voice became louder. He then began to appear very tense, grimacing and clenching his fists. When the primary nurse approached him, he seemed angry with her, and she was confused as to why.

The primary nurse reported her concerns to her head nurse: "I'm not sure what's going on with Mr. Anno, but I feel somewhat frightened of him." The head nurse paged Mr. Anno's physician and attempted to get a Spanish language interpreter to come quickly to the unit.

Mr. Anno's postoperative wound needed checking, so both the primary and head nurse approached the patient's bedside. Much to their surprise, Mr. Anno began shouting loudly, attempted to pull out his IV line and catheter and appeared to jump out of the bed. He picked up a wound dressing kit that was on his overbed tray and threw it at the head nurse. It hit her in the face, stunning her but not hurting her.

The two nurses then intervened appropriately in the following manner:

- *The head nurse announced that she would take charge.*
- *A call for help from the rest of the unit's staff was made, and one of them was told to notify the security staff.*
- *The other patients were removed from the area.*
- *The head and primary nurse and two nursing aides (one man and one woman) held Mr. Anno by his hands and feet.*
- *Another nurse brought some mechanical soft restraints, and under the head nurse's direction, these were placed on the patient.*
- *Mr. Anno's physician arrived, and after reviewing the situation, quickly ordered the following: Haloperidol 5 mg IM STAT to be followed by Haloperidol 5 mg IM every hour, until sedated.*
- *The patient was told in Spanish about the medication and why he would receive it.*
- *A staff member remained at the patient's bedside.*

After this incident was under control, the head nurse, primary nurse, physician, and the two nursing aides spent 20 minutes in a conference room reviewing the episode. A plan was made to confer with the family about Mr. Anno's mood swings, request a psychiatric evaluation, use Spanish-speaking personnel when available, and maintain close observation of this patient.

SUMMARY

Never underestimate the potential for violence. Nurses can be assaulted by a patient their size or larger, someone young or old. Incidents of workplace violence occur in every health care setting. The way nurses can avoid a potentially violent situation is to be prepared beforehand. They need to understand de-escalation skills and learn how to manage patients who become aggressive, before it occurs. In-service education and training about the health care institution and the unit's plan for such an emergency cannot be over-emphasized.

The best way to deal with a violent patient is to defuse the incident during the early stages of escalation. Nurses need to watch for early warning signs and try to avoid a dangerous outburst. When this fails, their own safety and that of other patients and staff members, as well as that of the aggressive patient, must be considered.

It is important that all nurses have some education or training in safe and appropriate use of precautions to follow for these untoward and least expected episodes.

EXAM QUESTIONS

CHAPTER 10

Questions 57-61

57. A factor that may increase the risk of a workplace violence incidence is

    a. distraught family members.
    b. working in a team.
    c. the entrance to hospitals controlled by security.
    d. the employment of primarily experienced staff.

58. An early warning sign of a violent episode may be when a patient

    a. is quiet and withdrawn.
    b. is hysterical laughing and agitation.
    c. has elevated lithium levels.
    d. is yelling, teeth clenching, and angry appearance.

59. The general recommended number of staff members needed to restrain a patient safely is

    a. one to two.
    b. two to four.
    c. five to six.
    d. eight to nine.

60. Common *DSM-IV-TR* disorders associated with violent patients are organic mental syndromes, substance abuse disorders, and

    a. obsessive-compulsive disorders.
    b. bipolar affective illnesses.
    c. schizophrenia.
    d. paranoia.

61. Nursing responsibilities related to managing patients who are or have the potential for workplace violence is to

    a. encourage patients to express anger verbally rather than "acting out."
    b. get close to the patient to indicate you have control of the situation.
    c. avoid the use of stress reduction techniques until the patient has calmed down.
    d. observe patients who are potentially dangerous once a shift.

CHAPTER 11

NURSING MANAGEMENT OF THE NONCOMPLIANT PATIENT

CHAPTER OBJECTIVE

After completing this chapter, the reader will be able to recognize the major risk factors for noncompliance by patients and specify interventions to increase compliance.

LEARNING OBJECTIVES

After studying this chapter, the reader will be able to

1. describe noncompliance and the health belief model.
2. discuss risk factors associated with noncompliance.
3. list the NANDA nursing and *DSM-IV-TR* diagnoses related to noncompliance.
4. identify nursing interventions that may be used when caring for noncompliant patients.

INTRODUCTION

The concept of noncompliance is a subject of debate in health care. Nurses have argued that the diagnosis of noncompliance labels the patient negatively. It places the emphasis on the patient's behavior instead of on a mutual process with the nurse. At issue is the right of the patient to choose a treatment course that is different from the recommendations of the health care team.

Compliance is usually associated with optimal health. The most obvious result of noncompliance is that the disorder may not be relieved or cured. For example, when patients fail to take their prescribed medications it can lead to optic nerve damage and blindness in people with glaucoma, to an erratic heart rhythm and cardiac arrest in people with heart disease, and to stroke in people with high blood pressure. Failing to take prescribed doses of an antibiotic can cause an infection to flare up again and may contribute to the emergence of drug-resistant bacteria (Hussar, 2003).

Dealing with patient noncompliance may present some of the most difficult and, at the same time, rewarding experiences for nurses.

DEFINITIONS

What is *noncompliance*? The NANDA (2003) definition of noncompliance is:

"Behavior of a person and/or caregiver that fails to coincide with a health-promoting or therapeutic plan agreed on by the person (and/or family and/or community) and health-care professional. In the presence of an agreed-on, health-promoting or therapeutic plan, person's or caregiver's behavior is fully or partially nonadherent and may lead to clinically ineffective or partially ineffective outcomes."

This definition recognizes the change that has occurred in the past 25 years from medically directed treatment regimens to an emphasis on the patient as an active consumer and decision maker.

The nurse's role as advocate and facilitator for patients and families negotiating health care systems is a pivotal one. The difference between compliance and noncompliance may be due to the relationship between the nurse, the nurse's interventions and the patient.

Another definition is that the term "compliance" is used to describe the degree to which patients follow their health care providers' recommendations. It implies a patient-health care provider hierarchy, or a power differential in the relationship, in which the patient is relegated to a subordinate role. Some health care professionals believe this has a negative influence on patient compliance with the health care provider recommendations (Schroy, 2002).

Health care professionals use their power as a means to control and manipulate their patients. Health care professionals also reward compliant patients. Rewards that a nurse might give to a compliant patient may include a smile, more time spent in the patient's room, or a quicker response to the patient's call light. If asked, many patients state that they are afraid that if they do not behave in a certain way, the nurse will "retaliate."

In order to promote compliance, hospitalization must become an experience in which patients maintain control over most of what happens to them. Providers are finding new ways to alleviate the dilemmas that patients face when hospitalized. An example is the PCA pump for self-administration of pain medication. Use of this device reduces the patient's dependence on the nurse for comfort and, in many cases, reduces anxiety about pain control.

INCIDENCE

According to an estimate from the Office of the U.S. Inspector General, drug therapy noncompliance results in 125,000 deaths from cardiovascular disease each year, up to 23% of nursing home admissions, and 10% of hospital admissions (Hussar, 2003).

Estimates of the extent of noncompliance vary widely. Studies over the past three decades have shown that patient noncompliance with treatment regimens can range from 20% to a staggering 80%, depending on the kind of treatment (Jaret, 2001). It is estimated that on average patients follow doctors' advice correctly only about half of the time, and when a treatment regimen is complicated or difficult, for example, lifestyle changes to control hypertension or diabetes, compliance is even lower (Jaret, 2001).

HEALTH BELIEF MODEL

Many attempts have been made to create a conceptual model of compliance that will enable health care providers to predict and understand patients' behavior. The Health Belief Model (HBM) offers some understanding of the phenomenon of compliance. The model proposes reasons for people's varied and unique responses to illness. The significance of this model is that a patient's choices depend on his or her beliefs and not necessarily on the medical evaluation of the situation.

The health belief model proposes that changes in beliefs about the severity of and susceptibility to, a health outcome and its consequences are associated with the motivation to take action. Once an individual feels threatened, a decision is made among alternative actions based on a cost-benefit analysis.

The model postulates that people choose health actions when they are faced with a threat to their health. The actions they choose depend on three perceptions (Clemens-Stone, et al., 2002):

1. The perceived susceptibility of the health threat.
2. The perceived severity of the health threat.
3. Perceived benefits if preventive action is taken. What the cost will be in their lives if they take the recommended health action.

For many patients, noncompliance may be their perception that the illness is less of a problem than the treatment is.

LEGAL AND ETHICAL ISSUES

Health care professionals are faced with increasingly complex situations in which the patient's wishes may deviate from the treatment recommendations. Some ethical guidelines can help nurses choose a response to a patient who is noncompliant. In addition, to practice within the law, nurses must be aware of legal guidelines. This area of health care is changing quickly. Nurses need to be clear about their obligations to patients and be knowledgeable about patients' rights.

Rights of the Patient

Inviolability is the fundamental right of every individual to be left alone. The U.S. Constitution and Bill of Rights are based on this principle. The individual should have authority over what happens to his or her body. In practice, however, the situation is not always so clear. In some instances, individual rights may interfere with the rights of others. In addition, fluctuations in public sentiment may affect the decisions made by practitioners and institutions.

Ethicists differ on their perceptions about the dilemmas that health care professionals face. The concept of personal freedom becomes unclear when the perspective is one of social responsibility. Some ethicists believe that people can have both individual autonomy and responsibilities to one another.

The issue of mandatory testing for communicable diseases illustrates the dilemma of conflicting principles. Inviolability would guarantee the individual the right to refuse such testing. The principle of social responsibility would support mandatory testing, because the individual has the obligation to participate to protect others.

Legal Concerns

One legal issue that affects nursing when discussing patient compliance is the issue of competence. A patient is considered competent if he or she is able to participate in making decisions, which means the patient has the ability to comprehend information, understand their choices and communicate his or her decision verbally or nonverbally to the health care team. For example, patients must be able to understand the nature of their illness and the treatment alternatives available. Equally important is an understanding of the consequences of any decision the patient might make about these alternatives.

Patients are presumed to be competent. This assumption means that the burden of proving incompetence belongs to parties other than the patient. Unless otherwise indicated, we assume patients are making competent choices about their health care.

At times, however, patients may be caught in a frustrating contradiction between the issues of compliance and competence. A patient may refuse a treatment recommendation. Health care professionals may label the patient incompetent because of the refusal. In this situation, a cognitively capable patient has made an informed decision. However, because the patient has made the "wrong" decision, health care professionals view him or her as incompetent.

Special Cases

Rights of pregnant women

Pregnancy offers a unique slant to the issue of patients' rights. For some people, the fact that the fetus is affected by the mother's behavior alters the mother's right to personal freedom. The legal system has increasingly overridden the right of the pregnant mother to disregard medical advice.

The legal basis for these decisions is weak. However, societal support for protecting the unborn fetus can result in disregard for the rights of the pregnant woman. The current debate over the rights of the unborn fetus versus the rights of the mother evokes intense emotions on both sides of the issue.

Withholding nutrition

There is little consensus on the ethics of withholding or withdrawing nutrition from patients. When a patient chooses to refuse nutrition, it is often difficult for health care providers to honor this wish. Nurses may be concerned about participating in behavior that will lead to hunger or thirst in the patient. The American Nurses Association (ANA) holds the position that the decision to withhold artificial nutrition and hydration should be made by the patient or their surrogate after consultation with the health care team.

In some ethical deliberations, a distinction is made between allowing a patient to die and killing a patient. The difference lies with the intent of one's actions. Nutrition may be withheld on the premise that, if given, it will prolong life and thus prolong suffering. This is different from starving a patient with the intent to kill him or her. Others argue that the finality of the act of withholding nutrition makes the act untenable.

It is imperative that every nurse be familiar with the legalities surrounding patients' right to refuse treatment. In addition, careful thought concerning the nurse's own ethical position on these issues is necessary. The answers are not always clear in the increasingly complex environment of health care today.

The Patient Who Signs Out Against Medical Advice

Leaving the hospital against medical advice (AMA) may be an extreme example of noncompliance. It is rarely a spontaneous act. There are often warning signals or repeated conflictual interactions with staff members before the patient actually signs out.

Nurses and physicians alike react strongly when a patient leaves AMA. Health care providers may attempt to cajole or coerce the patient into staying, since there are often concerns about the patient's safety and the providers' obligations to the patient.

Patients should be free to leave AMA as long as they are competent and not endangering their life. It is not appropriate to medicate a nonpsychotic patient who is threatening to leave AMA. Using drugs as chemical restraints in this manner is questionable from a legal standpoint.

RISK FACTORS

Noncompliance has meaning in the patient's life. The nurse must be able to carefully assess the patient's situation to understand this meaning. In this way, obstacles to compliance can be uncovered and dealt with. Patients' individual characteristics and living conditions will influence the likelihood of them being compliant or noncompliant. Knowledge of risk factors can help nurses be more aware of the possibility that a patient may have difficulties following their treatment plan. This knowledge is most helpful when it is used to prevent possible problems with compliance.

Psychological and Cognitive Risk Factors

The most important psychological risk factors include the following:

- Cognitive abilities
- Mental status
- Denial and anxiety
- Addictions
- Depression
- Past experiences

Psychological and cognitive factors influence compliance. To be able to comply, patients must understand the information presented to them. Teaching should be brief and focused. Complex information should be broken into smaller and more understandable parts whenever possible. It is helpful to simplify teaching material as much as possible.

Patients with cognitive deficits may not be able to learn. Patients must have an adequate attention span to be capable of concentrating and learning new behaviors.

Similarly, patients with changes in mental status may be unable to integrate new learning material effectively. Their judgment may be significantly impaired. A thorough mental status examination is needed if there is any indication that a patient's mental status is compromised.

Some patients may be in denial, a defense mechanism used to guard against uncomfortable feelings. They may be too frightened by their illness to be able to accept it. This can cause them to feel their treatment recommendations are unnecessary. They need time to adjust and an opportunity to discuss these difficult feelings.

Denial is a normal part of grieving and sometimes occurs in people when they find out they have a terminal illness. Illness and hospitalization involve losses for people regardless of the prognosis, and denial may be part of any patient's presentation.

Anxiety reduces anyone's ability to process information or to make decisions. An anxious patient might behave in a number of ways, including anger, complaining, demanding, withdrawing, or even crying. When a patient's anxiety is reduced, it will aid in them being compliant with their treatment regimen. Many patients are fearful of the unknown. Education often allays these fears.

Addictions affect compliance because drugs take top priority in the addicted person's life. If the treatment regimen interferes in any way with the addictive behavior, the patient will not be compliant until the addiction is treated. The classic example of this is the alcoholic who has cirrhosis. The recommended treatment is abstinence from alcohol, but few alcoholics can accomplish this without professional intervention.

Depressed patients are 3 times more likely to be noncompliant with medical treatment recommendations than patients who are not depressed (DiMatteo, et al., 2000). A person who is clinically depressed will not take in information or make decisions as well as one who is not depressed. Depressed persons have low self-esteem and feelings of hopelessness that can interfere with their ability to follow a regimen to better their health. It is the most common mental health problem in the United States. Unfortunately, although it is probably the easiest to treat, it is the least treated and depressed patients are often overlooked.

Finally, each patient enters the health care system with ideas and beliefs that affect the course of the current hospitalization. Previous experiences that were negative can affect a patient's expectations. If a patient enters the system expecting the worst, chances are good that health care recommendations will not be viewed in a positive light.

Age

The estimated rate of noncompliance for elderly people is 50%. They are more at risk for noncompliance than other adult patients. Because of their unique needs, older patients present a challenge in compliance. Their hearing, vision, and cognitive functioning are likely to be impaired in some way. These handicaps make changes in behavior difficult.

Most patients age 60 and older require correction of vision. These impairments make self-administration of medications particularly difficult. Almost one-third of all people ages 65-79 have significant hearing impairment. In elderly patients, recall is best when material is given verbally. Information must be delivered slowly and audibly.

Depression is common in elderly patients. It often goes undetected and untreated. Depression lessens the ability of older patients to adapt to changes in their lifestyle. Seemingly, simple tasks such as picking up a pill become difficult. Plans for self-treatment must take this loss of dexterity into account.

Older people often find that their social support systems are shrinking. Friends and relatives may be ill, dying, or making changes in living arrangements. This resulting isolation can affect compliance.

The number of medications prescribed for older patients can be a problem. At least one-fourth of elderly patients recently discharged from hospitals have six or more prescriptions that require self-administration.

It is easy to see why the noncompliance rates for elderly patients are high. This population is also less likely to be assertive about their needs with health care providers. Elderly patients constitute a major part of general care patients today. Nurses need to be sensitive to the unique needs of this age group.

Social-Economic Risk Factors

The social spheres that most affect a patient's health behaviors are as follows:

1. Family, significant others
2. Relationships with health care providers
3. Cultural or ethnic group
4. Religious community or beliefs
5. Economic status

Patients are more likely to comply with their treatment plan if their family or significant others are supportive of it and encourage them to follow it. They are also more likely to be compliant if they have a positive relationship with their health care team, are included in the decision-making and acknowledged for being compliant.

A patient's cultural or religious beliefs and practices may prohibit compliance with a treatment regimen. Some religions view the use of certain types of medical interventions as a lack of faith in God, and those procedures are therefore prohibited. Some cultures have lay healers, and the patient may wish to combine the healer's cures with medical treatment. Many cultures view healing as a family affair; therefore, the family will need to be always present and involved in the patient's care. Nurses must try to understand and appreciate the importance of these practices in order to help patients be compliant.

A significant concern related to noncompliance is limited income. Patients may have hospitalization coverage but few funds to follow through on recommendations after discharge. A patient who must choose between feeding his or her family and buying blood pressure medicine has no choice at all. It is helpful to examine patients' finances with them and planning realistic health care choices together.

Environmental Risk Factors

The health care setting can influence patient compliance. The most common factors seen here are comfort issues and ease of access, including transportation. The needs of physically impaired patients must be considered carefully. For example, an elderly person who has been directed to return to the clinic after a surgical admission may not keep this appointment. The patient may not have transportation, the parking may be too remote for them to comfortably walk from the car to the building, or the stairs may be too much for them to handle. If there is little to motivate the patient's return, these environmental obstacles will result in noncompliance.

Determining risk factors early in treatment enables nurses to intervene effectively. Nurses are in the best position to use their skills to develop a care plan with the patient that maximizes compliance. In the same way, knowledge of risk factors affecting compliance can enhance discharge planning and make if more effective.

Situational factors are best dealt with through anticipatory planning. A conversation with the patient about the possibility of these events occurring and how to deal with them can ensure their compliance. A patient on a restricted diet, for example, is asked to consider eating at home until he or she is familiar with the diet. The patient is also given ideas about what to order in a restaurant that would be allowed on this diet. The patient may feel uncomfortable explaining their diet to friends. Role playing situations such as these can be helpful.

DSM-IV-TR DIAGNOSES

- Noncompliance with Treatment

Can be seen in the following *DSM-IV-TR* diagnoses

- Delirium, dementia, and other cognitive disorders
- Substance-related disorders
- Mood disorders
- Anxiety disorders
- Schizophrenia and other psychotic disorders
- Eating disorders
- Personality disorders

NANDA NURSING DIAGNOSES

- Noncompliance*

Related diagnoses include the following:

- Anxiety
- Ineffective coping
- Compromised family coping
- Deficient knowledge
- Powerlessness
- Self-care deficit

THE NURSE'S REACTION TO THE NONCOMPLIANT PATIENT

Nurses' willingness to examine their attitudes and feelings is of primary importance in dealing with noncompliant patients. The identity of nursing is closely tied to the concepts of helping, caring, and service. When a patient appears to reject a nurse's expertise in promoting wellness, the nurse must deal with many intense and conflicting emotions.

Many nurses state that they would prefer to spend their time with motivated patients who want to get well rather than with a patient who does not comply with his or her treatment plan. They express anger that the patient is "wasting" a bed, precious resources, or nurses' time.

* most common

Sometimes, this anger leads to withdrawal of services to that patient. A nurse may avoid going in the patient's room or omit teaching the patient, because "the patient isn't going to do it anyway."

At times, nurses may feel unable to "allow" a patient to be noncompliant. This situation might occur when the nurse has some commonality with the patient, such as being the same age as the patient or having a parent who died of the disease the patient has. Nurses who feel powerless in the face of a patient's noncompliance may push the patient to comply while assuming decision-making responsibilities that belong to the patient.

Depending on the reasons for the noncompliance, the patient may be quite happy to be left alone or to be overly dependent on the nurse. More likely, however, the patient recognizes that his or her real health care needs go undetected. This behavior may become a cycle. (Table 11-1.)

TABLE 11-1: CYCLE OF NONCOMPLIANCE BETWEEN PATIENT AND NURSES
Noncompliance Cycle
• Patient is noncompliant
• Nurse feels angry, powerless, and so forth.
• Nurse withdraws or becomes overactive
• Patient's needs go unmet
Nursing Strategies to Stop This Cycle
Nurses:
• Becoming aware of feelings
• Performing a nursing assessment
• Using care planning as a mutual process

INTERVENTIONS

- **Intervention:** Develop awareness of your feelings toward patients who are noncompliant with their treatment regimen.

  Rationale: If you are unaware of how you feel toward noncompliant patients, you may be unaware that you are feeling angry, and/or powerless toward a noncompliant patient. You may withdraw from the patient and his/her needs will go unmet.

- **Intervention:** Develop a trusting relationship with your patients.

  Rationale: Trust is basic to a therapeutic relationship. The quality of the nurse-patient relationship has been shown to be a powerful predictor of adherence.

- **Intervention:** Assess your patients' mental status.

  Rationale: Several studies have shown that clinical depression is a risk factor for noncompliance.

- **Intervention:** Explain clearly why the treatment is necessary and what to expect (e.g., delayed benefits, general side effects).

  Rationale: A complicated or demanding treatment plan is an ordeal for even the most motivated patients. Patients need to understand why the plan is necessary; otherwise, they have little incentive to follow through with it.

- **Intervention:** Include the patient in setting goals and planning care.

  Rationale: The mutuality of expectations of patients and nurses makes it more likely that patients will be compliant with the treatment plan. Encourage patients to ask questions and express their concerns regarding their illness and the advantages and disadvantages of a treatment regimen.

- **Intervention:** Teaching should be aimed at the patient's learning level.

  Rationale: To be able to comply, patients must understand the information presented to them:

  - Teaching should be brief and focused.

- Complex information should be broken into smaller, more understandable parts whenever possible.
- Teaching material should be simplified as much as possible.

- **Intervention:** Encourage patients to report problems with their treatment regimen, such as any unwanted or unexpected effects, before adjusting or stopping it.

  Rationale: Patients often have valid reasons for not following a treatment plan. The better you understand your patients' concerns about their treatment regimen, the more likely you will be able to explain its importance.

- **Intervention:** Encourage patients to request the help of family or friends.

  Rationale: If family members or other caregivers are not providing direct care to patients, and if patients are having difficulty following through on taking medications or other therapies, family members can be helpful in reminding patients to take their medications.

- **Intervention:** Communicate your concerns about the patient's noncompliance with other members of the health care team.

  Rationale: The health care team may detect and help solve noncompliance problems.

CASE STUDY

Mr. Scovil is a 60-year-old man who was admitted to the hospital after he fell and broke his hip. He had been helpless at home for several hours after the fall, because his wife was at work. On the day of admission, surgical repair was performed with the insertion of a nail and plate.

After surgery, Mr. Scovil was disoriented for several days. He was confused and belligerent and had visual hallucinations, and physical restraint was required part of this time. His blood pressure and pulse rate were high.

When his mental status cleared, his physical progression through the postoperative period was smooth. The incision healed with no excessive redness or swelling. His vital signs became stable.

However, it was difficult to develop a pain management regimen that enabled Mr. Scovil to experience pain relief. He was unwilling to practice coughing or deep breathing as ordered. It was a constant struggle to get him to ambulate, although he had been taught the dangers of immobility many times.

His wife and children rarely visited and were unwilling to talk with staff members. Mr. Scovil reported that he had not worked for many years and relied on his wife financially. He gave vague reasons for this situation, stating that he had been laid off and that there were never any jobs in his field of construction.

The nursing staff began to be concerned as time passed and Mr. Scovil did not appear to be assuming responsibility for his recovery. He, on the other hand, was eager to return home and pressured his physician to let him go prematurely. The staff called a patient care conference to discuss the discharge plans for Mr. Scovil.

During the conference, several of the nurses on the evening shift expressed concern that Mr. Scovil would not be well taken care of if he were to return home at this time. They had met his wife because she visited in the evening after work. They described her as "cold" and "mean." They were sure that she would provide no assistance to Mr. Scovil, who would be forced to fend for himself at home.

The night nurses described ongoing episodes of insomnia that the patient had experienced since his admission. One of the nurses had found Mr. Scovil attempting to smoke in his room. She stated that he drank cup after cup of coffee whenever he could. They thought that he was simply a noncompliant patient and should be discharged as soon as possible with home care assistance.

One of the nurses mentioned the possibility that Mr. Scovil might be alcoholic. She cited his delirious episode after admission, his low pain tolerance, and the dysfunction in the family as possible indicators that he might have a substance abuse problem. The physician added that the hypertensive episode after surgery and the insomnia supported that assessment.

The social worker remembered that Mr. Scovil's wife had bitterly discussed with her his lack of employment and his numerous falls. The social worker admitted that she had focused on the wife's hostility instead of on the possibility of alcoholism. She added that the behavioral habits of smoking and excessive coffee drinking have been linked to alcoholism.

It was agreed that the social worker would meet again with Mrs. Scovil and discuss the possibility that Mr. Scovil was an alcoholic. With the information from that interview, it was easier to approach Mr. Scovil about his problem and he was in fact referred for treatment of a substance abuse problem.

The evening staff nurses who described the patient's wife as cold and mean were clearly angry. If they had examined their feelings closely, they might have discovered that they were actually angry with the patient for his unwillingness to participate in recovery. It is often easier to be angry at a healthy, and distant, family member than to be angry with the patient. It can be difficult for nurses to accept their anger at a patient who is ill and with whom they interact on a daily basis.

The night nurses felt little compassion for this patient. They were most likely dealing with feelings of powerlessness. Mr. Scovil was a patient who ignored the rules and the health care advice offered to him. Powerlessness is difficult for anyone to feel and is most often masked by anger and rejection.

Most of the issues of noncompliance in this case study were attributable to the untreated chemical dependency. Mr. Scovil was unable to be compliant because of this addiction. If he were discharged home without treatment of this problem, his chances of a successful recovery would have been low. In addition, his alcoholism would have placed him at risk for more falls and other physical problems.

SUMMARY

Noncompliance is an emotionally laden issue for many health care providers. The noncompliant patient presents a unique challenge in patient care. Social, environmental, and psychological risk factors are associated with noncompliant behavior. Knowledge of a patient's risk factors is helpful in preventing potential problems with compliance.

Nurses should be willing to examine their own feelings about patient noncompliance. A patient who appears to be rejecting treatment recommendations can evoke many conflicting emotions. Nurses must be aware of these feelings, in order to have therapeutic interactions with patients and help them with noncompliance problems.

EXAM QUESTIONS

CHAPTER 11

Questions 62-68

62. Which model postulates that patients choose noncompliant health actions based on their perception that the illness is less of a problem than the treatment?

    a. Health belief.
    b. Health actions.
    c. Predictors of noncompliance.
    d. Illness perceptions.

63. The issue of mandatory drug testing is a good example of the ethical conflict of the

    a. rights of unborn fetuses versus rights of pregnant mothers.
    b. debate about the right to refuse treatment.
    c. rights of the individual versus the rights of society.
    d. debate about an individual's right to confidentiality.

64. A defining characteristic of a competent patient is a person who

    a. has not been coerced into making a decision.
    b. makes the right decisions for his or her health care situation.
    c. is oriented and alert.
    d. is physically and mentally able to participate in making decisions.

65. A common defense mechanism used by patients who are not compliant is

    a. projection.
    b. suppression.
    c. rationalization.
    d. denial.

66. An environmental risk factor associated with noncompliance is

    a. number of health care providers.
    b. limited income.
    c. transportation problems.
    d. church affiliation.

67. The most common nursing diagnosis associated with a patient who is not adhering to an agreed-on plan of care leading to a clinically ineffective outcome is

    a. noncompliance.
    b. deficient knowledge.
    c. powerlessness.
    d. self-care deficit.

68. In dealing with noncompliance, of the following nursing interventions, the best one the nurse has to affect a patient's behavior is

    a. acting mature.
    b. developing patience.
    c. self-awareness of feelings toward patient.
    d. developing a caring attitude.

CHAPTER 12

NURSING MANAGEMENT OF THE MANIPULATIVE PATIENT

CHAPTER OBJECTIVE

After completing this chapter, the reader will be able to recognize manipulative behaviors by patients and intervene appropriately.

LEARNING OBJECTIVES

After studying this chapter, the reader will be able to

1. recognize developmental patterns that may predispose the use of manipulation as a need-gratifying mechanism in adulthood.
2. list NANDA nursing and *DSM-IV-TR* diagnoses that have manipulative behavior as a feature.
3. identify criteria for nursing assessment of manipulative behavior.
4. discuss effective methods for intervening with manipulative patients.

OVERVIEW

The term manipulate means to get one's needs met indirectly, often at the expense of others, and often when a more direct expression of one's needs would be unsuccessful in achieving the desired result. The manipulator's goal is not only to get a particular need met but also to gain power over another person.

Illness poses a severe threat to a person's security, self-esteem, and autonomy. It results in a loss of self-control and a fear of becoming helpless and dependent. The health care system often further strips patients of a sense of control. The resulting anxiety may prompt a regression to manipulation as a coping mechanism even in patients who are not typically manipulative.

The stress of hospitalization may cause a patient to resort to manipulation in an effort to meet needs that he or she is usually able to meet independently. This anxiety-provoked regression may account for what is often perceived as an abundant use of manipulation among patients. It in turn evokes a negative response from nurses.

A DEVELOPMENTAL VIEW OF MANIPULATION

Before nurses can intervene effectively, they must understand not only what manipulation is and how they respond to it but also where it begins. How does manipulation become entrenched as a need-gratifying mechanism?

The use of manipulation as an adaptive need-gratifying mechanism starts early in life. The term adaptive maneuvering has been coined to describe the manipulative responses of newborns (Kumler, 1963). It is defined as an automatic behavioral pattern that a person adopts to decrease anxiety without learning or experiencing personal growth.

Newborns quickly and automatically learn several adaptive maneuvers to get their basic needs met. They manipulate without any regard for the needs of others. In newborns, who are utterly dependent on others, the use of manipulation is acceptable and, in fact, vital. It is a matter of survival.

As newborns grow and develop through childhood, they test a variety of adaptive maneuvers to manipulate the environment to gratify their needs. If a child's unacceptable experiments are met with clear and consistent limits delivered by primary caretakers with unconditional love and acceptance (of the child if not of the behavior), then the child will gradually develop a sense of self-esteem and self-control. Slowly, children learn to replace manipulation with more independent, adaptive behaviors.

If, on the other hand, a child's first limit-testing manipulative efforts are met with inconsistent limits or with no limits at all, with conditional love, and with lack of acceptance of the child, then the child will not learn how to fulfill his or her needs and how to gain love and acceptance from others.

ADAPTIVE MANIPULATION VERSUS MALADAPTIVE MANIPULATION

Manipulation is a behavior that we learn to use early in life. It is a process that occurs consciously or unconsciously in virtually all-interpersonal interactions.

When manipulation is used in an adaptive sense, it is just one of a wide repertoire of behaviors that a person can call on to ensure that his or her needs are fulfilled. It is neither the only need-gratifying behavior nor the dominant one.

For the manipulation to be considered maladaptive, it will depend on:

- The extent to which it is used as a dominant need-gratifying mechanism
- The degree to which a person is aware of using it
- The degree to which the person is self oriented, not oriented to others
- The degree to which others are treated as objects
- The effect on others, for example, leaves the person who was manipulated feeling angry but not necessarily certain about why.

Unquestionably, the word manipulator has taken on a pejorative connotation. However, the fact is that we all manipulate at times as a way of ensuring that our needs are met.

It is important to understand that isolated uses of manipulation do not make a person a manipulator.

IDENTIFYING THE MANIPULATOR

Health care professionals may overuse the term manipulative. Nurses may be prone, after a difficult day or after caring for a string of particularly taxing patients, to assign the label manipulator to the patient who makes that one final demand that sends them over the edge, or to the patient who is just a little too insistent in his or her self-advocacy. If the term manipulative is to have clinical meaning, its characteristics must be understood.

Manipulators are not always easy to recognize.

They are often charming, entertaining, and intelligent. They rarely see themselves as having a problem and are unlikely to seek help on their own. In fact, many manipulators are loathe to change their behavior even when confronted with the reality of it, because it gets their needs met.

When the harmful effect on others is pointed out, manipulators may feign guilt or remorse, because they are aware that these are the socially acceptable responses. But they will not actually feel these feelings. Manipulators do not have a superego (concerned with moral behavior) strong enough for pangs of conscience to be genuine. The reaction of the nurse faced with such a situation is, understandably, negative.

Thus begins the cycle of manipulation

A person has needs to be met but cannot trust the environment to meet them consistently. The ensuing anxiety causes the person to fall back on the earliest need-gratifying mechanism-adaptive maneuvering and manipulation-to ensure that his or her needs are met. If the manipulation is effective, the anxiety temporarily decreases. Success! The person's needs have been met. However, the pattern of manipulation has been reinforced.

When the same person gets a negative response, he or she becomes angry and frustrated, and anxiety skyrockets. The person again tries desperately to manipulate in an effort to regain control. The pattern is set.

Lacking basic trust, the person is caught in an endless cycle of having to manipulate in order to ensure that his or her needs are met-in order to survive. In the process, though, the person is likely to alienate all those around him or her, who soon learn that they cannot trust the person. The issue of developing trust, then, is key. The manipulative patient-one who uses manipulation maladaptively-has little concern for the wants and needs of other people. Because manipulators do not trust their own feelings, they cannot trust others. This lack of trust leads to a sense of loss of control, and the manipulator tries to regain a sense of self-mastery by controlling others.

THE NURSE-PATIENT CYCLE OF MANIPULATION

The manipulative patient is uncannily adept at seeking out others' unique weaknesses and vulnerabilities and using those weaknesses and vulnerabilities to gain control. Their manipulative behavior can be active or passive.

Active manipulation may involve any of the following behaviors:

- Making demands: "I want my medication at 9 o'clock, not 8 o'clock. I don't care about your rules!"
- Violating rules and routines: Everyone has to be back from a day pass by 6 o'clock. "Forget it! I'm going out with my friends. I'll get back when I'm good and ready."
- Making threats: "If you don't get that guy and his obnoxious family out of my room this minute, I'm going to tear up this place and you along with it!"

Manipulative behaviors can also be passive, and subtler:

- Eliciting pity: "Can't you understand how hard it's been for me lately? My husband is leaving me for another woman, my two kids are out every night until 1 a.m., and my son wrecked a brand new car last weekend. Wouldn't you drink too?"
- Ingratiating and flattering: "You're the only one on this unit who can possibly understand me. I don't even know why you're working here-you're so much smarter than the rest of them. And prettier too."
- Evoking guilt feelings: "Well, if you had come in here to talk to me at 2:15, when you said you would, I wouldn't have gotten so depressed, and I wouldn't have had to cut my wrist."
- Abusing compassion: "You said you understood how hard it was for me to be in this hos-

pital, so I was sure you'd understand why I needed to sneak out this morning. I'm back now, so take it easy. Why do you have to search me? You said you trusted me!"

- Attempting to exchange roles and become the helper's helper: "I heard you tell one of the nurses that you're having trouble with your son. I can't believe he doesn't appreciate having a mother like you. I'm about his age, I'll bet. Tell me what he's doing. Maybe I can help."
- Pitting staff members against each other: "I couldn't get that other nurse to understand why she should persuade the doctor to discharge me tomorrow. She said not to discuss it with you because you're too new to understand the rules yet. But I know you understand my situation. Will you explain it to my doctor? And pick a time when she's not around to interfere."
- Questioning competence or authority: "My doctor said that I could have another sleeping pill if the first one didn't work. Can't you even read a chart? Well, you're not in charge around here anyway. We'll see what happens to your job when the nursing supervisor comes in tomorrow."

In each of the foregoing examples, the patient seized on a particular need of the nurse (the need to be professionally competent; to maintain a safe, consistent environment; to be viewed as empathic and understanding) and geared his or her behavior to exploit that Achilles' heel, that window of vulnerability.

When nurses realize they have been successfully manipulated, their likely response is a range of negative feelings and behaviors, including anger, frustration, indifference, and withdrawal. Although manipulative patients will enjoy these responses as signs of their power, they will also feel an inward sense of increasing anxiety, because once again they have successfully managed to manipulate someone. Can no one be trusted? Will no one ever be able to see through them and give them what is truly needed-a sense of realistic limits and a genuine feeling of self-control?

Figure 12-1 illustrates the vicious cycle of manipulation that can play out repeatedly between nurse and patient when manipulative behaviors are not accurately diagnosed and nursing interventions are not put in place to halt the cycle.

If nurses are to stop the cycle, self-awareness is vital. If they have difficulty with their own self-

FIGURE 12-1: THE NURSE-PATIENT CYCLE OF MANIPULATION

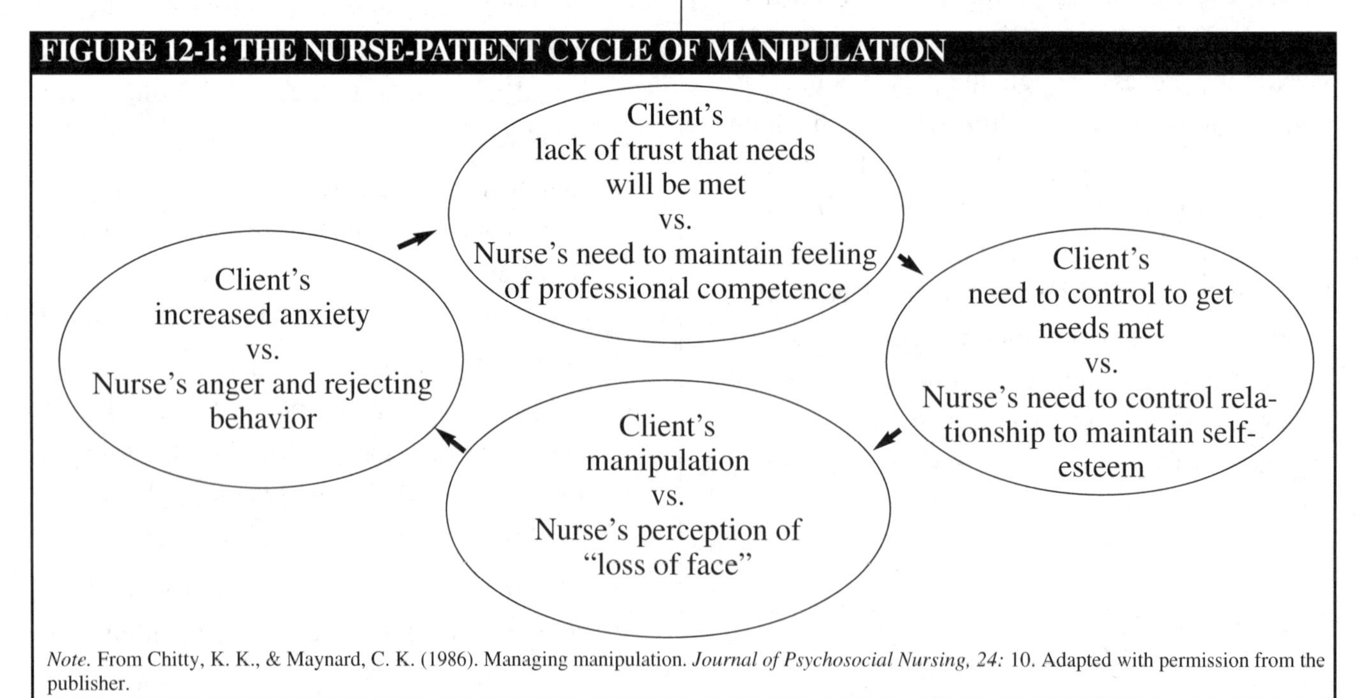

Note. From Chitty, K. K., & Maynard, C. K. (1986). Managing manipulation. *Journal of Psychosocial Nursing, 24:* 10. Adapted with permission from the publisher.

esteem, they will be vulnerable to manipulative behavior. The key is for nurses to be aware of their needs so they will know when they are being exploited. They also need to be aware of their own responses-of their feelings of anger, need to withdraw, frustration, and loss of objectivity-as indicators that they are being manipulated. Only then can they be effective in helping patients find more adaptive ways of getting their needs met.

DSM-IV-TR DIAGNOSES

As noted earlier, manipulation is ubiquitous. Nurses may encounter manipulation in any patient, on any unit, in any circumstance. However, some *DSM-IV-TR* diagnoses are more likely than others to have manipulativeness as a characteristic. They are:

- Conduct disorders
- Eating disorders
  - Anorexia nervosa
  - Bulimia nervosa
- Factitious disorders
- Personality disorders
  - Antisocial personality disorder
  - Borderline personality disorder
  - Dependent personality disorder
  - Histrionic personality disorder
  - Narcissistic personality disorder
- Substance-related disorders

DSM-IV-TR diagnoses provide good preliminary clues to manipulation. Any nurse assigned to a patient with one of the diagnoses in this list should be on the alert for manipulative behavior. However, it would be an error to rely on the *DSM-IV-TR* diagnoses as a sole indicator.

Many patients who have these diagnoses may not be maladaptively manipulative. The opposite is also true. Many patients who do not fit one of these diagnostic categories may use manipulation as a primary need-gratifying mechanism. Much more reliable then is a thorough nursing assessment.

NANDA NURSING DIAGNOSES

NANDA nursing diagnoses associated with manipulation most often has to do with nursing diagnosis: Powerlessness. Other nursing diagnoses are as follows:

- Impaired social interaction
- Ineffective coping
- Chronic low self-esteem
- Situational low self-esteem
- Fear
- Risk for loneliness

NURSING INTERVENTIONS

Manipulative patients are a difficult nursing challenge. Patients may be unable and unwilling to recognize their manipulative coping mechanism. Even when the nurse points it out, the patient may not be willing to change. As noted previously, manipulation is inherently rewarding. However, manipulation also has a way of alienating others and of making it impossible for the patient to form meaningful relationships. The nurse who can help manipulative patients recognize the effects of their behavior and find alternative need-gratifying mechanisms will do much to improve the patients' quality of life.

The following interventions may be useful.

- **Intervention:** Establish a trusting relationship.

  Rationale: Establishing a trusting relationship is as difficult as it is vital.
- Deception is a way of life for the manipulative patient, but every other intervention will be

based on the foundation of a trusting nurse-patient relationship.

- It may be the first trusting relationships that the patient has ever had in his or her life. Allow time for trust to develop.
- **Intervention:** Recognize the problem and determine who generates it.

  Rationale: Patients cannot be helped to find more adaptive ways of living if they do not recognize their current behavior as a problem, and take responsibility for the circumstances in which they find themselves.
- **Intervention:** Provide a consistent environment.

  Rationale: Inconsistent caretaking is at the root of the development of maladaptive manipulation as a coping mechanism in early childhood.
  - The goal of manipulation is to somehow make the environment safe and secure.
  - Knowing what to expect decreases the manipulative patient's anxiety and helps him or her learn to trust others and the environment.
  - In addition, consistency reduces the patient's opportunity to divide the staff by manipulating them.

  Formulate long- and short-term goals. To ensure that every member of the staff carries out the treatment plan as consistently as possible-vital to ensuring that the patient cannot manipulate by "splitting" the staff-all team members should have input into setting goals.

  The short-term goals are that the patient will do as follows:
  - Recognize and verbalize feelings of anxiety, frustration, or powerlessness.
  - Recognize instances of manipulative behavior.
  - Gain insight into the effect of manipulative behavior on others.
  - Distinguish between wants and needs and learn to delay immediate gratification of both.
  - Verbalize acceptance of responsibility for own actions.
  - Limit manipulative behavior and determine and practice alternative methods for gratifying needs.

  The long-term goal is that the patient will determine and express needs and desires in a clear, direct manner that does no harm to others and that demonstrates responsibility for the patient's own actions.
- **Intervention:** Refuse to respond to manipulation.

  Rationale: Refusing to support the manipulative behavior tells manipulative patients that you cannot be used as an object. They will have to find another way of getting you to meet their needs.
- **Intervention:** Do not accept the behavior, but accept the patient.

  Rationale: Manipulative patients are in desperate need of acceptance and positive regard. Try to get yourself—and the patient—to recognize the patient's behavior as manipulative rather than label the patient as a manipulator.
- **Intervention:** Help the patient to understand the impact of his or her behavior on others.

  Rationale: Do not assume that empathy comes naturally to manipulative patients.
  - Help them develop an awareness of their impact on others by being honest about your own feelings.
- **Intervention:** Set reasonable, clear, firm, consistent limits (Table 12-1).

  Rationale: Although patient will rail against limits, they will be enormously relieved by them.

TABLE 12-1: TEN STEPS TO SETTING LIMITS WITH MANIPULATIVE PATIENTS
1. Define clear expectations.
2. Communicate expectations positively and firmly.
3. Limit only those behaviors that clearly impinge on the well-being of the patient or others.
4. Make sure that the limits are in the patient's best interests and are not punitive.
5. Offer a brief rationale for the limit, but do not engage in a debate about its fairness or justification.
6. Define the consequences of exceeding the limit—and make sure that they are consequences that you can carry out.
7. Hold all discussions related to limit setting on a one-on-one basis, in private. (This limits the opportunity for the patient to involve an "audience" in determining whether the limit is "fair" or not.)
8. Make sure that all staff members understand the limit and its consequences as they were communicated to the patient.
9. Stand firm in the face of the inevitable testing of the limit.
10. Provide positive reinforcement each and every time the patient is able to meet the limit.

- They will provide the external control patients need until they can develop internal control.

- **Intervention:** Help the patient develop and practice alternative methods for gratifying needs.

  Rationale: Manipulative patients will be loath to give up a successful need-gratifying mechanism if they do not have another one with which to replace it.

- **Intervention:** Provide positive reinforcement every time the patient is able to
  - Communicate a need directly,
  - Take responsibility for himself or herself, or
  - Accept a limit.

  Rationale: The patient needs to recognize not only unacceptable behavior but also acceptable behavior.

  - Reinforcement of positive behavior is likely to elicit more positive behavior.

SUMMARY

The manipulative patient is among the most difficult of nursing challenges. Nurses may be well aware of the patient's desperate need for help and must get past a myriad of negative emotional responses of their own in order to give that help.

EXAM QUESTIONS

CHAPTER 12

Questions 69-74

69. Manipulation is
    a. always a sign of poor mental health.
    b. develops during the turbulence of adolescence.
    c. always conscious.
    d. a behavior that everyone uses at one time or another.

70. Maladaptive manipulation
    a. ends when the need is met.
    b. is mutually determined by both parties.
    c. leaves the person who was manipulated feeling angry but not necessarily certain about why.
    d. can be growth producing.

71. At its most basic level, the development of manipulative behavior is a failure to
    a. develop trust.
    b. develop a sense of guilt.
    c. develop love for one's caretakers.
    d. experience anxiety.

72. An example of a *DSM-IV-TR* diagnosis that gives a good preliminary clue to the potential of a patient being manipulative is
    a. anorexia.
    b. adjustment disorder.
    c. psychotic disorders.
    d. schizophrenia.

73. According to the objective criteria for a nursing assessment of manipulation, the following scenario describes a manipulative patient:
    a. At 10:45 a.m., for the second time, Mr. J. approaches the nurse's station for his 10:00 medications.
    b. The nurse observes Mr. B. hiding his medication under his pillow. He denies having done it and reminds her that he is the King of France.
    c. The nurse finds a bottle of whiskey in Ms. M.'s drawer. Ms. M. immediately admits to having hidden it there and is genuinely remorseful.
    d. Knowing that an important radiograph was scheduled for today, Mr. M. leaves the unit. He laughs when, on his return, the nurse reminds him that it is against policy to leave the hospital without informing the staff and that he missed a very important test.

74. An example of a well-set limit is

 a. Unit policy states that alcohol is not permitted in patients' rooms. Please get rid of that bottle now, or I will have to call security.
 b. You're always having too many people come up to visit you. No more visitors for the rest of the week.
 c. Everyone has to attend physical therapy. If you don't go, you can't have your medication at 2:00.
 d. Mr. A. brought a bottle of alcohol up to the unit, and that's against the unit's policy, so Mr. A. will not be permitted to have visitors for the rest of the week. Don't the rest of you think that's fair?

CHAPTER 13

NURSING MANAGEMENT OF THE PATIENT WITH CARDIOVASCULAR DISEASE

CHAPTER OBJECTIVE

After completing this chapter, the reader will be able to recognize common psychological responses to acute cardiovascular disease, and those that occur in recovery phases.

LEARNING OBJECTIVES

After studying this chapter, the reader will be able to

1. specify behaviors seen in patients before cardiac disease develops, during the acute illness, and in the recovery phase.
2. list NANDA nursing and *DSM-IV-TR* diagnoses related to coronary artery disease.
3. describe the characteristics of near-death experiences.
4. discuss family responses to the acute illness of a loved one.

INTRODUCTION

Persons at risk for coronary artery disease (CAD) share many common physiologic and psychosocial behavior traits. No one trait causes CAD, but the combination of traits increases the likelihood of developing the disease. Some traits cannot be changed, but most can be modified to decrease the risk of CAD. This chapter briefly reviews psychological risk factors. It goes beyond pre-CAD assessment to include common responses of patients and their families to critical cardiovascular diseases and to the discharge and rehabilitation phases of CAD.

BEHAVIORS BEFORE CAD

In addition to the physiologic risk factors for CAD, some psychological behaviors are common in persons in whom cardiac disease develops. Friedman and Rosenman (1974) have called these behaviors type A or coronary-prone behaviors. They contrast this behavior with type B behavior. In reality, few persons are purely type A or type B. Most have combinations of behavior styles but tend to lean one way or the other. Some behaviors are learned while the person is growing up; some develop later. None are so much a part of the personality that they cannot be changed. However, change can be difficult and requires a real commitment to be successful.

Type A behaviors (refer to Table 13-1) typically occur in achievement-oriented persons who work with great intensity, aggression, and urgency to accomplish tasks. These people tend to struggle to fit more and more into less and less time. A type A person is always rushed, impatient while waiting, and has difficulty letting others finish their thoughts or sentences. Type A persons expect oth-

TABLE 13-1: TYPE A PERSONALITY CHARACTERISTICS

- Achievement oriented
- Difficulty letting others finish their thoughts or sentences
- Extremely competitive
- Always rushed
- Possess a strong sense of urgency
- Check their watches frequently
- Often obsessed with their work
- Will do almost anything to accomplish their goals
- Work with great intensity, aggression, and urgency to accomplish tasks
- Impatient while waiting
- Vague guilty feelings during periods of relaxation
- Tend to struggle to fit more and more into less and less time
- Expect others to share this intensity and to make the same commitments
- More likely to get heart disease
- If they have heart disease, they are more likely to diligently follow their treatment plans

ers to share this intensity and to make the same commitments. The feeling of time urgency makes it difficult for type A persons to take time to be creative and leads them into stereotyped behavior in which they cannot accept change.

This achievement orientation is not limited to work; it extends into family relationships and the few outside activities that type A persons permit themselves. They may demand high achievement from their children in school, or expect to be always on the winning team, or to own the best car or home.

Type A persons frequently ignore their psychological and physiological needs. They tend to internalize their feelings, and often have problems with low self-esteem and self-worth, and have excessive dependence on the approval of others.

Any nurse who works with type A persons needs to understand their intense behavior patterns. Recognizing stress as a major risk factor of CAD is important. Telling patients to "decrease stress" will be futile. Patients must really believe that a stress reaction is harmful before they will attempt to change their behavior.

Patients who have chest pain during an intense business meeting might be able to correlate stress with heart disease. Patients may believe that they are at risk if others in their peer groups, who share the same lifestyles, have heart attacks or must have cardiac surgery. Patients who have asymptomatic CAD will be the hardest to convince.

Patients who do relate their stress reactions to heart disease may have one or more responses. Those who perceive heart disease as a realistic threat to their lives may be motivated to make lifestyle changes.

However, the changes often are temporary because the patient reverts to a previous coping style. Denial of illness or total major restriction in activity are opposite ways that persons use to cope with a threat to their body image. A diseased heart cannot be seen and therefore can be denied. Others are frightened by this threat and restrict all activity thereby becoming cardiac invalids.

Threats to self-image (the way a person sees himself or herself in relation to social and work roles) may make a person feel changed in an indescribable way. A patient may feel that he or she is no longer a competent provider or spouse, is not the same dynamic leader at work, or is useless and in the way.

BEHAVIORS DURING THE ACUTE ILLNESS

Shock and Disbelief

During the acute phase of cardiac illness, patients generally experience a normal grief response. The most common response to cardiovascular disease such as myocardial infarction is denial. Patients have a host of explanations for their signs and symptoms: indigestion, a pulled muscle, toothache, and so forth. They rationalize these manifestations by saying, "This cannot be happening to me. I just had a complete physical." Or, "I don't think my heart is the problem. Let me out of here."

It is important that people are aware of this reaction and act quickly to obtain needed medical help. In the hospital setting, nurses need to know how the patient describes the symptoms: for example, "pressure," "indigestion," "arm pain," or "chest pain." A patient who is experiencing intense substernal pressure may give a negative response to a question about chest pain and thus delay treatment.

While denying the severity of their illness, the patient also experiences fearful thinking "What is happening to me," "Why can't I stop this pain," or "Am I dying?" This stage of shock and disbelief lasts a few minutes to a few days.

During the period of denial, it is important that the nurse allow this defense mechanism. Denial in the first hours and days of illness protects the patient from anxiety and fear. Anxiety and fear will increase the release of catecholamines, increase the myocardial workload of an already compromised heart, and thus promote further damage to the heart. Arguing with a patient in denial also increases the release of catecholamines and cardiac activity.

Nursing actions need to support reality but not force it on the patient. Patients who will not believe that their heart is the problem and who want to be released from the ICU can be told, "I know it's hard to believe your heart could be the problem. Just to be sure, we need to keep you here for a few days to check blood tests and ECGs, which will give us the answer. How can I make your time here more comfortable?" Fear during this stage can be minimized with calm, truthful explanations and frequent bedside interactions. Sedative medications may be useful also, but they never should be used in place of interpersonal communication.

Development of Awareness

When patients start to realize that something is wrong with their heart, they are becoming aware. In this stage, they move in and out of anger, bargaining, and depression. Anger may be directed at themselves or others, with comments such as "I did what my doctor said, but I still had a heart attack. What kind of doctor is he?" Or, "Why didn't I stop smoking earlier?" Or, "You don't let me sleep. No wonder I'm sick!"

Bargaining usually is done with a higher power or authority. It is not unusual to hear a patient say, "If I only live through this, I'll go to church regularly." Or, "If I get better, I'll stop smoking." Bargaining may be done through patients wishing to see a clergy member. Bargains with physicians and nurses are usually long-term proposals (e.g., I'll quit smoking if I live through this) and need little intervention other than active listening. Short-term deals (e.g., I'll take my medicine if I can walk to the bathroom) should be addressed on an individual basis. A good approach is to do whatever will decrease the myocardial workload.

Depression is common 3-5 days after a myocardial infarction. This is a time when the physiological signs and symptoms usually have resolved, and the focus turns to what has happened to the patient and how it will affect the patient's life. Feelings of powerlessness and low self-esteem are common: "I can't do anything now. What good am I as a husband (or wife)?"

Depression can be a source of concern to family members who now see the patient improving physically and cannot understand the patient's failure to feel positive. It is important to explain to both the patient and the patient's family that this is a normal stage of recovery. To help move patients through depression, increase their activity as soon as possible. Use a firm, kind approach to maintain the patient's self-respect as you get the patient up and bathed. Specific directions such as "walk to the next doorway and back 3 times each day" are more helpful than "gradually increase your activity." Depression that lasts longer than 1 week may require psychiatric intervention.

As patients enter the period of developing awareness, the nurse should understand that their anger is not a personal attack but rather a way to release frustration and energy. Remember that many patients who have myocardial infarction are type A personalities who cope with stress by trying to get control over the situation, and who are impatient with anything outside of their usual activity of schedules. Anger may be expressed in words or in actions (e.g., pulling off ECG leads, climbing over side rails, or refusing treatments).

The nurse should avoid arguing with the patient, but should set limits so patients will not harm themselves or others. Sometimes giving patients more control over their situation helps decrease anger and increase compliance. Letting the patient who is on bed rest sit in a chair may increase the patient's feeling of control, decrease anger, and consequently decrease the response of the sympathetic nervous system that otherwise would increase myocardial workload.

DSM-IV-TR DIAGNOSES

The psychiatric diagnoses that may be related to CAD are

- Major depressive disorder
- Brief psychotic disorder
- Psychotic disorder
- Delirium
- Generalized anxiety disorder
- Primary insomnia
- Acute stress disorder
- Adjustment disorder with depressed mood
- Sleep disorder

NANDA NURSING DIAGNOSES

The NANDA nursing diagnoses that are related to CAD include

- Anxiety
- Impaired adjustment
- Disturbed body image
- Acute confusion
- Defensive coping
- Ineffective coping
- Ineffective denial
- Grieving
- Hopelessness
- Noncompliance
- Acute pain
- Powerlessness
- Situational low self-esteem

ICU PSYCHOSIS

Intensieve Care Unit (ICU) psychosis occurs to some extent in the majority of ICU patients within 2-5 days of their admission to the unit. Because the patients' usual behaviors and usual state of health are not known to the ICU staff, some of the subtle behavioral changes that precede the more obvious psychosis may be missed.

Characteristics of ICU psychosis are impaired intellectual function, difficulty in judging reality, and an altered emotional state in a high-stress situation. Behavioral manifestations may include the following:

- Having auditory and visual hallucinations (hearing and seeing things not present)
- Misinterpreting stimuli (e.g., confusion about health care personnel in scrubs who are interpreted as business persons inappropriately attired in pajamas)
- Talking with people not present (e.g., family, spirits)
- Having feelings of persecution, especially related to painful or frightening procedures (e.g., suctioning, insertion of IV lines, moving into a scanner for computed tomography)
- Pulling at tubes and wires and possibly doing self-harm
- Trying to get away from perceived danger by climbing out of bed

Factors that promote ICU psychosis include the following:

- Disturbed sleep cycles
- Absence of a day-night cycle
- Frequent contact with the many staff members for care
- Hearing staff members who are on rounds talk about the patients in the unit
- Proximity of other patients with their inherent odors, noises, and activities
- Multiple pieces of equipment within the line of vision
- Meaningless noises of machines
- Lack of usual sensory stimulation
- Sedation, which blurs consciousness
- History of psychiatric illness or of drug or alcohol abuse
- Prolonged cardiopulmonary bypass

Treatment of ICU Psychosis

If admission to an ICU is anticipated (as occurs with patients who have cardiac surgery), preoperative teaching can help minimize the patient's confusion. Patients need to know that confusion and frightening dreams are common and do not indicate a psychiatric problem. They should be encouraged to discuss their fears before the operation and to share their feelings afterward.

Unplanned admission to the ICU adds another stressor for the patient. An accurate and thorough assessment is crucial, because differential diagnosis of psychosis is difficult.

To minimize ICU psychosis, decrease unnecessary stimuli. Turn off suctioning machinery when it is not in use. Move equipment out of the patient's line of vision. Turn off lights at night. Explain what the patient does see and hear, including resuscitation efforts, insertion of IV lines, multiple infusion pumps, multiple personnel, and teaching rounds. Keep the patient oriented to the environment, ICU personnel, time, and current events. Explain all procedures before performing them. Be truthful about uncomfortable procedures so patients know that you do not mean to hurt them. Involve the family in the patient's care if they desire. Simple activities such as applying a cool cloth to the patient's head can be comforting to both the patient and the patient's family.

If ICU psychosis does occur, continue activities to minimize it. Use simple and concrete explanations when talking to the patient. Do not agree with hallucinations, but do not belittle the patient. Statements such as the following do not take away the patient's self-respect, yet they promote orientation to reality: "I do not see those dogs that you see. I think they will go away as you get healthier." Support family members who may be frightened by the patient's bizarre behavior. Assure them that this is a temporary state and that it will pass.

Fortunately, ICU psychosis generally clears up after 24-48 hr on the regular nursing unit. Some confusion may take several days to resolve. Many patients do not remember any of the specific details of this period of time and need not be reminded. Patients' behaviors may be quite uncharacteristic and an unnecessary source of embarrassment for them.

Near-Death Experience

The near-death experience is a psychological phenomenon of persons who come close to death. Some studies suggest that up to 50% of persons who come close to death may have this experience. Many persons who have had a near-death experience are afraid to discuss it, thinking that they will be considered crazy. Others do not discuss it until many years after the experience.

Regardless of the person's age, sex, culture, religion, education, social class, or occupation, all near-death experiences have many common qualities. They are as follows:

- Separation from the body occurs. Persons can relate what actually happened to them during the time they were out of their bodies, describe people never seen before or since, and tell how they felt as the health care team worked to save their lives (some hoped not to be saved, and others hoped the resuscitation would be successful).
- Moving through a dark tunnel or space or through a fog is common. Many see a bright light on the other side that is associated with peace, love, and serenity.
- Many meet deceased relatives or friends, some of whom they may have had no knowledge of before the experience.
- Some meet a religious figure appropriate to their culture. This is not restricted to believers; it also occurs with nonbelievers.
- Persons see their lives pass before them or see significant people in their lives.
- Usually a sense of calm and relief from pain occur.
- Despite the pleasantness of the experience and the anticipation of pain on return, the persons understand a need to return to their body and do so.
- After the experience, persons have a sense of knowing about love and truth that they did not have before, and often they make lifestyle changes to promote this love.

Caring for a patient who has had a near-death experience requires sensitivity and patience. Even before you realize that a patient has had such an experience, you can help such patients by talking to them to keep them oriented about things going on during their unconscious period. Patients may be afraid to come right out and explain their experience for fear of being ridiculed. You can say that many persons who have been through a crisis like this have unusual experiences and leave an open-ended invitation for patients to talk about their own feelings.

It is important not to label near-death experiences as drug reactions or some psychopathologic response. Do not prod the patients; let them tell about their experience at their own pace.

Transfer Anxiety

A critically ill patient becomes dependent on the care of one or more nurses. Such patients are told that they are seriously ill, that they need total rest, and that they need to let others take care of them. They are attached to several machines that monitor all bodily functions, and, despite the discomfort of wires, they become comfortable with the fact that any problems will be noted immediately and be taken care of. If the moment of transfer from the ICU comes suddenly, patients may be fearful that they are being abandoned, and that something terrible will happen to them. This type of anxiety also can occur as care is transferred from one nurse to another within the ICU setting.

Transfer out of the ICU should be treated as a graduation or promotion to be eagerly anticipated, rather than a feeling of being dumped out for another patient's admission. In order to minimize transfer anxiety, it is important to prepare patients for the move. Show them how various monitoring devices are being removed as their health improves. Help them track their progress, for example, progressive ambulation, less IV medication to control chest pain, resolution of dysrhythmias, and healing of wounds. Give them progressively more responsibility for their care. For example, although a nurse could do the job more quickly, having patients bathe themselves gives them more independence and self-confidence.

Tell patients the expected length of stay in the ICU and where they will be cared for next. If possible, take them for a brief visit to the ward or step-down area before the transfer, or have the nurse from the ward see them in the ICU. At the time of transfer, introduce them to their new nurse (also applicable for shift-to-shift transfer within the ICU). This helps patients see that both nurses are part of the team and that care will be continued. If you promise to visit a patient after the transfer, keep your promise and do so.

Sometimes patients are transferred suddenly because a more critical patient is admitted. This should be avoided if possible, because the patient may not feel ready. Keeping patients informed of their progress and of the plans for their transfer will help decrease the anxiety associated with sudden transfers.

Coordination with physicians to transfer patients early enough to free beds for emergencies will help avoid the sudden transfer problem. If possible, visit suddenly transferred patients soon after the transfer to assure them of your interest in their welfare and of your coordination of their care with their new nurses.

HEART SURGERY

Deciding to Have Surgery

Deciding to have heart surgery is one of the biggest decisions many people make in a lifetime. The heart, the symbol of life, love, and courage, will be stopped, handled, cut, and sewn. No guarantee can be given that the operation will be successful or even that it will not be harmful. The patient will have to consider the possiblities of pain, prolonged recovery, financial expense, and possibly death.

Several factors can be helpful to consider for prospective cardiac patients and their families:

- Patients who view the surgery as giving them a new lease on life will approach the procedure positively. It is important that they do not believe that the operation is a cure for CAD or a magic potion that will make them younger.
- Patients need to be informed about complications, but they may focus more on life or death rather than potential long-term complications (e.g., stroke, bleeding, infection, heart attack).
- Patients generally are more concerned about the reputation and skill of their surgeons than about the reputation of the hospital.
- After the procedure, they are more attuned to the fact that most postoperative care is provided by the nurse, not the surgeons.

- The patient who perceives that the benefits of surgery outweigh the risks probably will consent to have the procedure.

Nurses play a major role with cardiac patients. The nurse needs to have a strong knowledge base about CAD, its available treatment options, and anticipated postoperative care. The nurse also needs to explore patients' feelings about their conditions with them and with their families.

Patients may have preconceived ideas about heart surgery from the positive and negative experiences of friends, popular magazines, television programs, fellow patients, or their own previous hospital experiences. They may have received medical information they did not understand. They may have unique concerns about family life, work, and finances after being diagnosed with CAD.

Whenever possible, a group approach to preoperative teaching is useful to help patients share common concerns and develop a support group. Such an approach is also more cost-effective and efficient for hospitals. Patients personal concerns can be addressed on an individual basis when needed.

After Surgery

Waking up after surgery can be a confusing experience. The patient has lost a big block of time while anesthetized and awakens with tubes running in and out of every orifice in the body. Although patients may appear to be awake, it may take several more hours until they are fully awake. If they have had good preoperative instructions, a simple explanation of what is being done will usually set their minds at ease. If the surgery was an emergency and no preoperative teaching was possible, the patient will need frequent explanations of care and restrictions.

Pain is usually a major postoperative concern. Many patients have no pain when lying still and only mild pain with activity. Others have significant pain while at rest and excruciating incisional chest pain with coughing and incisional leg pain with walking. The nurse should be aware of these variations in pain response and should give each patient adequate amounts of medication according to the patient's needs. The patient who is pain-free will be more relaxed and will cooperate more during treatments.

After the initial realization that they have survived surgery and have made it through 2 days of clinical progress, patients usually have a period of depression. This is similar to the depression seen in patients 3-4 days after a myocardial infarction. During this stage, patients cry easily, feel sicker, and have memory lapses. Patients who have been forewarned of this reaction usually have a less intense depression.

Going Home

Going home is a major milestone after heart surgery, but the joy is tempered by anxiety at leaving the security of the hospital. Spouses are also anxious because health care that was done by a professional team is being transferred to them. Like the transfer anxiety that occurs when moving from ICU to step-down or ward care, this anxiety can be minimized by good preparation, written instructions, and a telephone number to call for questions. Some hospitals have a nurse make a follow-up call to the patient's home the day after discharge to help ease the transition.

THE FAMILY'S RESPONSE TO CARDIAC ILLNESS

Families are an integral part of the patient's illness and recovery and need to be considered when care is planned. The acute physiologic needs of the patient are always of prime importance. Ideally, the patient's nurse will be able to care for the family, too. However, many times the staffing demands of the unit do not provide for an extended time with patients' families. In this situation, a social worker or a member of the clergy may be designated for family support. This should not be left for whomever is available; it should be a designated assignment for some member of the health care team.

When patients are critically ill, they are usually isolated from their families for extended periods. Events may have evolved rapidly, leaving family members disoriented and afraid that their loved one may die. Depending on their life circumstances and usual coping behaviors, family members may feel anger at the patient or the health care team for the illness, guilt that they did not encourage the patient to get treatment earlier, or depression and grief because of their stress.

Family members react to this stress in varied ways. They may minimize their loved one's illness to decrease the threat it imposes. Some intellectualize the illness by focusing on the technical aspects of care thereby blocking out their emotional responses. Some repeat information received or the sequence of events as if to convince themselves of their appropriate response.

Nurses need to be aware of the family's needs. Nursing research has determined the needs of families of critically ill patients, and overall the major one has been the need to have hope. Studies also have shown that often nurses did not rank family needs in the same order that the families did.

To most effectively care for the family, the nurse should take time to get to know each member, their past experiences, and their individual needs. Families should be encouraged to talk with the nurse, social worker, or clergy as well as among themselves. Verbalizing their fears and needs is usually more helpful than keeping silent about them. The nurse can provide privacy during brief family visits in the ICU; encourage hugs, kisses, or other signs of affection if desired; be available to a designated family member calling to get a report on the patient's condition; and convey their messages to the patient as this kind of tie to the family at home can be extremely therapeutic.

Once the critical illness is over and the patient is moved out of the ICU, families may be forgotten. Without frequent updates and progress reports, family members imagine all sorts of complications occurring. Keep patients and their families aware of progress to decrease their anxiety and prepare a smooth transition when discharge from the hospital occurs.

Homecoming for any cardiac patient may be met with a variety of emotions. The spouse may harbor suppressed anger at the patient for being ill, out of work, and shirking duties. The spouse may feel guilty if the illness occurred during sexual relations or when the patient was doing work for the spouse. Spouses often overprotect the patient, both as an expression of love and concern and out of fear that something will go wrong. Open communication in the hospital and at home is the key to minimizing homecoming anxiety.

RECOVERY BEHAVIORS

Recovery is a prolonged period that begins with discharge from the hospital and lasts for the rest of the patient's life. Patients may expect to return immediately to their previous level of activity, but find that they are weak, anxious, and depressed. They may have trouble sleeping because of a fear of dying. They may feel stifled by overprotection of their spouse, yet be afraid to be home alone. If they perceive their health as poor, they will have a slow return to normal life.

Family conflicts occur because of changes needed in diet, activity, and medications. Some patients may not be able to return to previous jobs or to do any work. Spouses and other family members may have assumed new roles in the patient's absence. Well-intentioned attempts to take over responsibilities and free the patient from pressures actually may diminish the patient's self-esteem and promote family conflict.

The nurse can prepare the patient and family for this recovery period by comprehensive teaching started several days before the patient's discharge. The patient and the patient's spouse should be present so they hear the same instructions and can ask questions. A group class is helpful for patients with similar problems so that families can learn from one another.

Patients and families need to know about anticipated emotional responses and to plan how they will handle these responses without hurting others. Instructions on diet, activity, and medications should be given. Spouses need to understand these instructions, but they should not nag competent patients to comply. Discharge orders need to be followed at home and the patient given the choice of following them. This puts the responsibility where it belongs, with the competent adult patient, and will minimize family conflict. Follow-up medical care also needs to be discussed.

Rehabilitation is a lifelong process. It is easier for patients to stay motivated if they have family and group support. Cooking prudent heart-healthy meals for the whole family increases compliance better than making one meal for the patient and another for everyone else. Exercise as a part of the daily routine and done with others is more successful than walking or exercising alone.

Formal groups for patients (e.g., Mended Hearts) and spouses are helpful for sharing concerns and for problem solving. The American Heart Association and the patient's hospital staff can suggest groups that meet patients and families' needs. A family physician that maintains close contact with the patient gives assurance of an interest in the patient's welfare and increases the patient's compliance.

SUMMARY

Psychological care of cardiac patients is a vital part of their recovery from illness. The heart symbolizes life, love, and emotions. Injury to the heart cuts to the very core of life and leaves patients and their families afraid of death or of radically changed lives. Comprehensive nursing care from the acute illness through recovery will help modify the psychological stress of cardiac illness and will promote full recovery for patients and their families.

EXAM QUESTIONS

CHAPTER 13

Questions 75-81

75. A type A person has just been told by a physician to cut back work hours to help decrease stress-induced hypertension. A typical response from this Type A person would be

    a. "I've been noticing a lot of pressure at work, and I planned to cut back."
    b. "I'm busy working on a big project. I need to work more hours, not fewer."
    c. "You're probably right. I'll give my biggest account to my partner to finish."
    d. "I'll just take a little nap after lunch and that will help with my stress."

76. To help minimize patients' anxiety at the time of transfer from the ICU to the ward, the nurse should

    a. keep them informed of their progress and the anticipated date of transfer.
    b. sympathize with them about the lack of good care on the wards.
    c. not talk about the transfer until it is happening so that you do not get their hopes up.
    d. tell them you will keep them in the ICU as long as possible so that they will be safe.

77. The patient says, "You don't know what you are doing! No wonder I'm not getting well faster!" The stage of grief the patient is in is

    a. bargaining.
    b. denial.
    c. anger.
    d. depression.

78. When patients are discharged from the hospitalized after cardiac surgery or treatment for cardiovascular disease, they usually feel

    a. ready to get back to work as soon as possible.
    b. glad to turn over their usual responsibilities to other family members.
    c. a renewed strength to get up and entertain visitors.
    d. frightened, anxious, and possibly, depressed.

79. Your patient says, "I don't think my heart is the problem. Let me out of here." The most appropriate nursing diagnosis is

    a. ineffective denial.
    b. noncompliance.
    c. acute pain.
    d. situational low self-esteem.

80. All near-death experiences have in common qualities, including

    a. moving through a dark tunnel or space; are psychotic.
    b. meeting a religious figure appropriate to their culture; have a mental illness.
    c. meeting deceased relatives or friends; always caused by a drug reaction.
    d. separation from the body occurs; see their lives pass before them.

81. Nursing research studies have determined that the major need of families of critically ill patients is to have

    a. hope.
    b. faith.
    c. security.
    d. information.

CHAPTER 14

USES AND ADMINISTRATION OF PSYCHOTROPIC MEDICATIONS

CHAPTER OBJECTIVE

After completing this chapter, the reader will be able to list the classifications of psychotropic medications and indicate the applicable nursing interventions for administering these drugs.

LEARNING OBJECTIVES

After studying this chapter, the reader will be able to

1. indicate which medications are antipsychotics, anxiolytics, antidepressants, and mood stabilizers.
2. discuss the psychiatric symptoms that may be relieved by antipsychotics, anxiolytics, antidepressants, or mood stabilizers.
3. recognize the potential side effects associated with the use of various psychotropic medications.
4. indicate nursing interventions used when administering psychotropic medications.

OVERVIEW

Nurses are legally and ethically responsible for knowing the psychotropic medications their patients are taking, including action, dosage, and adverse effects. They also need to be familiar with potential drug interactions of the medication they dispense to patients.

Psychotropic medications are prescribed for long- and short-term use and can be highly effective in treating the intended signs and symptoms of patients who are having emotional problems or who are mentally ill. A hospitalized patient may be beginning a course of a psychotropic medication (e.g., an antidepressant for the treatment of depression) or may already be taking a psychotropic medication to treat a mental illness and is hospitalized for an unrelated condition (e.g., diabetes). Some patients taking psychotropic medications may need to have their drugs discontinued temporarily while receiving other treatments (e.g., for surgery). The administration of these drugs should begin again when medically appropriate and ordered by the physician.

In administering psychotropic medication, the nurse should be prepared to teach the patient important information about the drug's action and potential side effects. Additionally, the nurse should be particularly observant for changes in the patient's mood and behavior to assess the effectiveness of these medications.

ANTIPSYCHOTICS

Antipsychotic medications (Table 14-1) are sometimes referred to as neuroleptics.

TABLE 14-1: COMMONLY PRESCRIBED ANTIPSYCHOTIC MEDICATIONS		
Generic Name	**Trade Name**	**Daily Adult Maintenance Dose Range (mg/D)**
TYPICAL ANTIPSYCHOTICS		
PHENOTHIAZINES:		
Chlorpromazine	Thorazine	50-1,200
Fluphenazine	Prolixin®	2-20
Fluphenazine decanoate Injection	Prolixin® decanoate	2.5-50 q 2-4 weeks
Mesoridazine	Serentil®	100-400
Perphenazine	Trilafon®	8-64
Thioridazine	Mellaril®	200-600
Trifluoperazine	Stelazine®	5-30
THIOXANTHENE		
Thiothixene	Navane®	5-30
DIBENZODIAZAPINES		
Loxapine	Loxitane®	20-100
BUTYROPHENONES		
Haloperidol	Haldol®	2-20
Haloperidol decanoate	Haldol® decanoate	50-300 q 3-4 weeks
DIHYDROINDOLONES		
Molindone	Moban®	20-100
ATYPICAL ANTIPSYCHOTICS		
DIBENZODIAZEPINES		
Clozapine	Clozaril®	25-900
BENZISOXAZOLE		
Risperidone	Risperdal®	0.5-8
THIENOBENZODIAZEPINE		
Olanzapine	Zyprexa®	5-20
DIBENZOTHIAZEPINE		
Quetiapine	Seroquel®	75-750
MONOHYDROCHLORIDE		
Ziprasidone HCl	Geodon®	40-160

Uses

Antipsychotics are considered safe, even when used in high doses. They are nonaddicting, produce no euphoria or tolerance and are not drugs of abuse. They are quite effective in decreasing some of the major signs and symptoms of psychosis.

Antipsychotics are prescribed to help stabilize a person's thoughts, behavior, and mood. Psychiatric symptoms that may respond to antipsychotic use include the following:

- Hallucinations
- Delusions
- Paranoia
- Catatonia
- Anxiety and agitation
- Hostility and rage
- Aggression and assaultiveness
- Disorganization of speech and behavior: flight of ideas, loose associations, illogical thinking, bizarre behavior
- Sleep disturbances

Antipsychotic medications may be used for prolonged periods, even years, either continuously or sporadically. They are helpful in relieving some of the clinical manifestations of acute and chronic psychosis. These manifestations include schizophrenia and related illness such as schizoaffective disorder. They do not cure schizophrenia but are generally effective in the treatment of altered thought processes associated with it. These drugs help a psychotic patient feel more normal and, therefore, better able to function. They also help patients who have schizophrenia better interact in psychotherapeutic treatment.

Neuroleptics are generally prescribed for short-term use for the following disorders:

- Anxiety disorders
- Brief psychotic disorder
- Mood disorders
- Organic brain syndrome with psychosis
- Substance-induced disorders

Action

Studies indicate that psychiatric disorders, including schizophrenia, psychotic disorders, mania, and substance-induced disorders, are related to increased dopamine activity. It is widely believed that antipsychotics work because they are postsynaptic dopamine antagonists. They block the neurotransmitter dopamine at the postsynaptic neuron receptor sites throughout the brain.

Since the early 1990s, newer antipsychotic medications or atypical antipsychotics, have appeared on the market. They offer effective treatment to many patients for which the older antipsychotic medications did not work. The newer drugs include Clozaril® (Clozapine), Zyprexa® (Olanzapine), Seroquel® (Quetiapine), Geodon® (Ziprasidone), and Risperdal® (Risperidone). These new antipsychotics offer hope to many people with chronic thought disorders, whose symptoms have been refractive to previous treatments.

Compared to typical antipsychotic, in addition to blocking dopamine receptors, the atypical antipsychotics also block serotonin receptors. This helps explain why atypicals are more effective in reducing signs and symptoms associated with psychosis and have fewer side effects.

The major classes of antipsychotics are as follows:

Typical

- Phenothiazines
- Thioxanthenes
- Dibenzodiazapines
- Butyrophenones
- Dihydroindolones

Atypical

- Dibenzodiazepines
- Benzisoxazole
- Thienobenzodiazepines
- Dibenzothiazepine
- Monohydrochlorides

It can take from several hours to weeks before the maximum antipsychotic effect of these medications occurs. Full improvement may take even more time be reached.

Choosing the right drug for each patient requires consideration of multiple factors. These include a patient's previous response to neuroleptics and the response of a blood-related family member, manifestations of the patient's illness, and the medication's side effect profile (beneficial or deleterious).

Side Effects

Nurses who are knowledgeable about signs and symptoms of both the patient's disease and potential side effects of their psychotropic medications can manage drug-induced problems at their earliest onset.

Antipsychotics differ in the severity and type of side effects they commonly produce. Each drug should be reviewed for its specific potential side effects before it is administered. The more common side effects of antipsychotic medications are usually not dangerous or severe, although the rarer side effects can be so severe as to be life threatening.

Many of the minor side effects are quite irritating, but accommodation usually occurs after a few weeks, and some side effects are diminished completely.

The following is a partial description of some of the more common side effects of antipsychotic medications (Stuart, 2002):

- *Anticholinergic:* These generally include dry mouth, blurred vision, constipation, vaginal dryness, nasal congestion, confusion, and decreased memory. Patients commonly complain of these side effects and often can accommodate to them. Urinary problems such as hesitancy or, more seriously, retention also can occur.
- *Cardiovascular:* ECG changes may occur with most antipsychotics. Orthostatic hypotension can occur, and patients may accommodate to it. The patient may experience fainting episodes and periods of light-headedness. This is common with the typical antipsychotics, Thorazine and Mellaril®, and atypical antipsychotic, Clozaril®. The nurse should assess patients for dizziness, syncope, and palpitations. The patient's vital signs should be monitored regularly. They should be cautioned to rise slowly from a lying to a sitting position before standing.
- *Skin reactions:* Patients can become photosensitive and thus need protection from the sun when outdoors. A rash can develop on the patient's trunk and back. The liquid-concentrate form of Thorazine can cause a contact dermatitis to the nurse who administers this medication.
- *Endocrine changes:* Menstrual malfunctions such as amenorrhea may occur, galactorrhea is seen occasionally, and some men may have gynecomastia. Sexual functioning and desire may be changed and limited.
- *Blood dyscrasias:* Agranulocytosis is a severe decrease in the number of white blood cells. Early signs and symptoms are sore throat, high fever, and mouth sores. If untreated, this can be life-threatening. It is a common side effect of Clozaril®, so patients taking this medication require weekly monitoring of their white blood cell count.
- *Neuroleptic malignant syndrome (NMS):* This is an idiosyncratic problem generally seen with the high-potency, long-acting medications, such as Prolixin® and Hadol®. This syndrome is similar to malignant hyperthermia. The patient has a change in consciousness, autonomic instability, moderate-to-high fever, and severe rigidity. Without treatment, neuroleptic malignant syndrome progresses rapidly; a decline in the patient's condition occurs within 12-24 hr. Because the signs and symptoms are generally insidious, this syndrome sometimes is not detected, and patients are thought to be having a worsening of their psychosis. An increase in the serum level of creatinine phosphokinase is one of the early confirmatory clinical indicators. NMS is clearly a life-threatening medical emergency, necessitating an ICU setting for monitoring and treatment. Nurses need to monitor their patients' temperatures, particularly, when administering high-potency antipsychotic medications.
- *Water intoxication:* This may develop over time with long-term use of antipsychotic medication. The patient consumes large quantities of fluid that results in sodium depletion.
- *Miscellaneous:* Occasionally seizures, abdominal distress, weight gain, jaundice, retinopathy, and hyperglycemia are seen.

Antipsychotic Medication-Related Movement Disorders

The Antipsychotic Medication-Related Movement Disorders are most commonly caused by typical antipsychotic medication, but also may be caused by some of the atypical antipsychotic drugs (Stuart, G.W., 2002).

- *Acute Extrapyramidal Syndromes:* Acute extrapyramidal syndromes are common in most patients receiving antipsychotic medications. They include dystonia, drug-induced parkinsonism, and akathisia.
- *Dystonia:* This refers to an acute dystonic reaction. It is characterized by involuntary muscle spasm, especially head and neck muscles. Sometimes the patient appears to be locked, fixed, or stuck in an uncomfortable position. The neck and face are affected in torticollis, the torso and back in opisthotonos, and the eyes in oculogyric crisis. Dystonic reactions are a true emergency and need immediate treatment, usually an injection of benztropine mesylate (Cogentin®) or diphenhydramine hydrochloride (Benadryl®).
- *Drug-Induced Parkinsonism:* This condition is referred to as pseudo-parkinsonism because it resembles Parkinson's disease. Symptoms include rigidity of muscles (arms most easily identified), slowed movements (shuffling gait), and tremor (more pronounced at rest). There is also a masklike face or loss of facial expression (blunted affect) present. It is treated with antiparkinsonian or anticholinergic medications such as Cogentin® and Artane®.
- *Akathisia:* This refers to a feeling of internal agitation or motor restlessness; the patient's legs will not stay still. Because this symptom is quite irritating, it may cause the patient to become noncompliant in taking their medications. It can be treated with Cogentin® or Benadryl®.
- *Neuroleptic Malignant Syndrome (NMS):* This is lethal side effect of antipsychotic medications. It typically develops 3-9 days after the administration of a high-potency antipsychotic medication. Symptoms include a fever (classic symptom), tachycardia, muscular rigidity, tremors, renal failure, impaired ventilations, muteness, and altered consciousness. Treatment is with dantrolene (Dantrium®) or bromocriptine (Parlodel®). If this condition develops, the patient's antipsychotic medication should be discontinued.

Chronic Syndrome

- *Tardive dyskinesia:* This is one of the more serious and prolonged of the extrapyramidal side effects. Patients who have tardive dyskinesia experience involuntary rhythmic movements of the mouth that include sucking, chewing, licking, and pursing movements. The tongue may protrude, and the face may be affected (such as, rapid eye blinking). A rocking like movement of the whole body also may occur.

If early signs of tardive dyskinesia are detected (through an Abnormal Involuntary Movement Scale examination), it is prudent to discontinue the current medication regimen. When high doses of antipsychotics are used, this side effect occasionally has an early onset. In other cases, the onset may be later, perhaps after many years of use and after a cessation of the medication. This side effect is sometimes irreversible if not detected early. Currently, no definitive treatment is available for tardive dyskinesia, although much research is being conducted to discover effective remedies for this syndrome. The best treatment is preventative measures using the lowest dose of medication with the nurse closely monitoring the patient for development of symptoms of tardive dyskinesia (Stuart, G.W. 2002).

Relief of Signs and Symptoms

Some antipsychotic medication side effects can be either beneficial or detrimental. An example is drowsiness. If a patient has been agitated, restless, and/or sleepless, this side effect would be beneficial. If a patient has had difficulty functioning or is fatigued and tired, drowsiness as a side effect would be detrimental.

As noted previously, the more common side effects of antipsychotic medications are generally effectively treated. Antiparkinsonian medications and antihistamines may produce acute relief of signs and symptoms for some problems associated with antipsychotics use. Benadryl® and Cogentin® are commonly given to reverse the discomforting problems of extrapyramidal side effects (EPSE).

Dietary changes may help with gastrointestinal and weight problems. Chewing gum or sucking candies can relieve a dry mouth. Stress reduction and physical activity can also be used when patients are preoccupied with some of the signs or symptoms.

Contraindications

Consideration should be given to the severity of the psychosis and the potential harm that may occur because of it (the traditional risk vs. benefit analysis). Some preexisting medical problems may require the complete cessation or avoidance of an antipsychotic. The following physical conditions should be ruled out before treatment with antipsychotics is started:

- CNS depression
- Blood dyscrasias
- Pregnancy and lactation
- Benign prostatic hypertrophy
- Previous allergic response
- Kidney and liver problems
- Glaucoma
- Cardiac insufficiency

ANXIOLYTICS

The anxiolytic drugs are also known as antianxiety agents or minor tranquilizers (Table 14-2). They are effective in producing a calming effect, a tranquil effect, and sleep.

In general, anxiolytics are safe. However, tolerance and psychological and physical dependence do occur over time. The daytime sedation effect must be monitored in active and fully functioning persons. Patients who use these drugs for a long time will go through withdrawal when the drug is stopped or the dosage is decreased. Such withdrawal may happen inadvertently in the general hospital if patients who are taking these medicines at home do not let the staff know at the time of admission.

These patients may become delirious, have severe episodes of anxiety and restlessness, have intense insomnia, or experience seizures. This possibility reinforces the need to obtain thorough drug histories from all patients. Instead of taking these medicines on an ongoing basis, it may be more beneficial for the patient to take them periodically for an acute problem and then discontinue them.

Uses

The main mode of action of benzodiazepine anxiolytics, such as diazepam (Valium) is generalized CNS depression. These medications enhance the effects of the inhibitory neurotransmitter gamma-aminobutyric acid (GABA).

The nonbenzodiazepines anxiolytic, zolpidem (Ambien®), acts on the benzodiazepine-GABA-BZ receptor complex, and shares some of the pharmacological properties of the benzodiazepines. The nonbenzodiazepines anxiolytic, buspirone (BuSpar®), controls anxiety by blocking the serotonin subtype of receptor, 5-HT1a, at the presynaptic reuptake and postsynaptic receptors sites (Stuart, 2002).

Benzodiazepine anxiolytic uses in clinical practice include the following (Stuart, 2002):

TABLE 14-2: COMMONLY PRESCRIBED ANXIOLYTICS

Generic	Trade Name	Daily Adult Dose Range (mg/D)
BENZODIAZEPINES		
Alprazolam	Xanax®	0.5-10
Chlordiazepoxide	Librium®	15-100
Clonazepam	Klonopin®	1.5-20
Clorazepate	Tranxene®	15-60
Diazepam	Valium	4-40
Halazepam	Paxipam®	80-160
Lorazepam	Ativan®	2-8
Oxazepam	Serax®	30-120
Prazepam	Centrax®	20-60
Temazepam	Restoril®	15-30
Triazolam	Halcion®	.25-0.5
NONBENZODIAZEPINES		
Buspirone	BuSpar®	15-30
Zolpidem	Ambien®	5-10

- Insomnia and sedation
- Relief from or lessening of anxiety
- Detoxification in treatment of drug addiction (Librium® or Ativan®)
- Muscle relaxation (Valium)
- Preoperative and postoperative sedation
- Anticonvulsants

Nonbenzodiazepines anxiolytics include the following:

- Zolpidem (Ambien®)—short-term treatment of insomnia
- Buspirone (BuSpar®)—generalized anxiety disorder—takes 2-4 weeks of continued use to be effective

The most common side effects associated with the use of benzodiazepine anxiolytics include the following (Stuart, 2002):

- Tolerance and addiction
- Daytime sedation and clouding of consciousness
- Impaired judgment
- Paradoxical agitation

Elderly patients seem to be particularly prone to some of these side effects, even though these medications often are prescribed for this age group.

Contraindications

Benzodiazepine anxiolytics should be prescribed with caution for the following patients:

- Known drug addicts, unless used in the medical management of a withdrawal regimen
- Patients with a compromised respiratory system
- Patients with severe liver damage
- Women who are pregnant or breast-feeding

Nonbenzodiazepine Anxiolytics Side Effects

Zolpidem (Ambien®)

- Abdominal pain, diarrhea, nausea, vomiting
- Abnormal dreaming
- Abnormal vision
- Amnesia
- Dry mouth
- Daytime drowsiness, fatigue, insomnia, lethargy
- Defective muscular coordination
- Depression
- Vertigo

- Headache
- Confusion (Spratto, Woods, 2003)

Buspirone (BuSpar®)

- Dizziness
- Headache
- Restlessness
- Drowsiness
- Nausea
- Nervousness
- Lightheadedness
- Excitement
- Abnormal or unwanted movements (Spratto & Woods, 2003)

Nonbenzodiazepine anxiolytics should be prescribed with caution if patients have liver and kidney problems.

ANTIDEPRESSANTS

Antidepressant medications (Table 14-3) are another category of commonly used psychotropic medication. They are used to treat major depressive disorder and depressions association with other disorders such as organic disease, alcoholism, and depressive phase of bipolar disorder.

The most widely prescribed antidepressants are tricyclic antidepressants (TCAs), monoamine oxidase inhibitors (MAOIs), and selective serotonin reuptake inhibitors (SSRIs). These medications elevate mood and alleviate other symptoms association with depression. They are effective in alleviating signs and symptoms of depression in 70-80% of cases.

The biochemical genesis of depression is fairly well accepted, partly because of the successful clinical results seen with the use of antidepressants. There seems to be a correlation between depression and the neurotransmitters norepinephrine, serotonin and/or dopamine. These biochemicals are stored in nerve cells and promote impulse transmission. When more neurotransmitters are available at the postsynaptic cleft, the signs and symptoms of depression seem to be fewer.

TCAs seem to increase the availability of neurotransmitters by preventing the reuptake of these biochemicals into the nerve cells. The neurotransmitters are not removed and so their concentrations within the synapse remain higher. SSRIs selectively block the uptake of serotonin. They do not bind with histaminic, cholinergic, dopaminergic, or adrenergic receptors, which result in producing fewer side effects than TCAs. MAO is an enzyme that metabolizes the neurotransmitters, and MAOIs prevent this metabolism. The result is an increase in the amount of neurotransmitters available for neuronal activity.

Tricyclic Antidepressants

TCAs have been in clinical use since the mid-1950s. Amitriptyline (Elavil®) and imipramine (Tofranil®) have been used as a mainstay of antidepressant treatment for more than 30 years.

Uses

TCAs are marketed specifically for the treatment of depression. The drug imipramine is also used in severe cases of enuresis in young children. A TCA introduced in 1989, clomipramine (Anafranil®), has shown good results in patients with obsessive-compulsive disorders.

With some exceptions, the TCAs generally require 2-3 weeks of continuous use before beneficial results are seen. Patients should be educated about this so they do not expect relief prematurely and thus think that they are not getting better, which can be discouraging or discontinue taking their medications prior to achieving therapeutic levels.

Side Effects

The specific side effects of TCAs vary somewhat from drug to drug and from person to person. The most common complaints and problems are the following:

TABLE 14-3: COMMONLY PRESCRIBED ANTIDEPRESSANTS

Generic	Trade Name	Daily Adult Dose Range (mg/D)
MAOIs		
Isocarboxazid	Marplan®	20-60
Phenelzine	Nardil®	45-90
Tranylcypromine	Parnate®	20-60
Reversible Inhibitors Of Monoamine Oxidase Type A		
Moclobermide	Manerix	
	Aurorix	
	Moclamine	300-600
Nonselective Reuptake Inhibitors		
Nefazodone	Serzone®	200-600
Venlafaxine	Effexor®	25-375
SSRIs		
Citalopram	Celexa®	20-50
Fluoxetine	Prozac®	20-80
Paroxetine	Paxil®	20-50
Sertraline	Zoloft®	25-200
TCAs		
Amitriptyline	Elavil®	
	Endep®	50-300
Amoxapine	Asendin®	50-600
Clomipramine	Anafranil®	25-250
Desipramine	Norpramin®	50-300
Doxepin	Adapin®	
	Sinequan®	50-300
Imipramine	Tofranil®	30-300
Nortriptyline	Pamelor®	50-150
Protriptyline	Vivactil®	15-60
Trimipramine	Surmontil®	50-300
Selective Presynaptic Noradrenergic Reuptake Inhibitor		
Reboxetine	Edronax	
	Vestra	4-10
Atypical Antidepressant		
Bupropion	Wellbutrin	
	Zyban	150-450

- Dry mouth
- Blurred vision, dry eyes, photosensitivity related to mydriasis (pupil dilation)
- Constipation
- Urinary retention or hesitancy
- Orthostatic hypotension
- Tachycardia and palpitations
- Sleep problems: insomnia or drowsiness
- Ataxia, unsteadiness, and tremulousness
- Weight gain or loss
- Paradoxical confusion, mania, or psychosis

Contraindications

TCAs must be used cautiously in patients who have cardiac conditions. A complete physical assessment and medical clearance should be obtained. Potential problems also should be considered in patients who have the following:

- Glaucoma, narrow angle
- Urinary problems, retention
- Benign prostatic hypertrophy
- Seizure disorders
- Impaired liver function

Caution: During the early stages of therapy with TCAs, suicidal tendencies can increase as the depression lifts and the patient now has the energy to kill them self. These drugs are a potent means with which to overdose. Close supervision by staff is imperative at this time.

Monoamine Oxidase Inhibitors

MAOIs have a long history of use with depression. They are also effective in the management of panic disorder and phobic disorders.

For some time now, MAOIs have been less popular because of the required dietary restrictions. Ingestion of foods containing tyramine can precipitate an acute hypertensive crisis. However, newer Reversible Inhibitors of Monoamine Oxidase Type A (RIMAs), such as Moclobemide (Manerix), are being developed. RIMAs agents are distinguished from MAOIs by their selectivity and reversibility. They are short-acting drugs and allow the recovery of enzyme activity in hours rather than weeks (Long, 2003).

Treatment with these newer drugs does not necessitate the special dietary restrictions required for MAOIs. Clients, however, should be advised to always take these drugs after meals and to avoid the consumption of excessive amounts of aged or overripe cheese and yeast extracts in order to minimize tyramine potentiation and the possibility of a hypertensive reaction (Long, 2003).

With the older MAOIs a tyramine-free diet must be followed to avoid the danger of a hypertensive crisis. Some of the foods to be avoided include the following:

- Aged cheese
- Red wine
- Bananas, avocados
- Salami, sausage, dried fish, liver
- Caffeinated coffee, tea, colas
- Beer
- Chocolate
- Yeast products
- Yogurt
- Pickled products
- Soy sauce

Additionally, some medications can cause the same problem, including Ritalin® (methylphenidate), Demerol® (meperidine), and most of the over-the-counter cold and diet preparations.

Nurses who care for patients who are taking MAOIs should review with them a complete list of foods and medications to be avoided. In addition, MAOIs and TCAs should not be given together, except under rare, closely monitored situations.

Side Effects

Possible side effects associated with the use of MAOIs include the following:

- Dry mouth
- Constipation
- Blurred vision
- Orthostatic hypotension
- Urinary problems
- Edema
- Confusion

Contraindications

Use of MAOIs should be avoided in patients who are considered unreliable or who cannot maintain the dietary restrictions. Patients should be assessed medically, and use of these antidepressants avoided if there is evidence of the following:

- Liver and kidney disease
- History of stroke or cardiovascular disease
- Hypertension
- Hyperthyroidism
- Seizure disorders
- Pheochromocytoma
- Glaucoma

Selective Serotonin Reuptake Inhibitors

SSRIs exploded onto the market in the late 1980s with the introduction of Prozac® (fluoxetine) for the treatment of depression. This drug, as well as its successors, is highly effective in the treatment of depression.

Patients may experience relief from the signs and symptoms of depression generally after 3-5 days of use, compared with 10-14 days for the TCAs. Steady state plasma levels are attained after 4-5 weeks of continuous drug administration (Spratto & Woods, 2003). An additional benefit is the milder side effects. Like TCAs, SSRIs can cause a manic episode. Therefore, patients taking these inhibitors should be monitored for any changes in behavior. Another potential side effect is acute aggressive reaction, which could necessitate discontinuance of the medication.

Side Effects

- Dry mouth
- Blurred vision
- Urinary hesitancy
- Constipation
- Insomnia
- Agitation
- Headache
- Orthostatic hypotension
- Weight loss
- Sexual dysfunction: in men: abnormal ejaculation or impotence; in women: delay or loss of orgasm (Spratto & Woods, 2003; Stuart, 2002)

Contraindications

Serotonin syndrome: Caused by concurrent use with MAOIs—and other drugs that increase serotonin, such as tryptophan, and amphetamines.

Symptoms include:

- Mental status changes
- Restlessness
- Myoclonus
- Hyperreflexia
- Seizures
- Tachycardia
- Hypertension
- Diaphoresis
- Tremors
- Shivering
- Ataxia or incoordination
- Headache (Sternbach, 2003)

MOOD STABILIZERS/ ANTIMANIA MEDICATIONS

Lithium Carbonate

Lithium carbonate (Eskalith®, Lithobid®, Lithonate®), a mood stabilizer, is used primarily as the drug of choice in the treatment of manic episodes of bipolar disorder. Patients who have been initially stabilized with lithium may need to take it long term.

Lithium is an element, rather than a substance synthesized in a laboratory. A specific concentration of lithium in the blood must be maintained to produce stabilization of a patient's mood disorder. The specific mechanism of action for lithium carbonate and how it works in stabilizing manic and depressive episodes is unknown. Lithium may enhance the reuptake of norepinephrine and serotonin, thus decreasing the levels in the body and stabilizing mood.

The behavior and thought processes of manic patients can change markedly once lithium therapy is started. After taking this medication for 7-10 days, patients may have a dramatic improvement in their manic behavior.

The daily lithium adult dosage range for acute mania is 900-1,800 mg. which is adjusted to obtain serum concentrations between 0.8 and 1.2 mEq/L (in blood samples drawn before the patient has had his first lithium dose of the day). The maintenance daily adult dosage range of lithium is 300-1,200 mg. to achieve serum concentrations between e 0.6 and 1.0 mEq/L. The dose range of lithium has a narrow margin of safety, since symptoms of lithium toxicity begin at serum blood levels of 1.5 mEq/L and greater (Long, 2003).

The patient's blood sample is obtained and analyzed 12 hr after the patient's last dose of lithium. Initially, blood levels may be monitored two or more times each week. After a patient has been stabilized, one time each month is generally adequate. The frequency of monitoring can be decreased as use of lithium progresses from initial titration to long-term maintenance.

Regardless of specific dosage, there is a cause-and-effect relationship between lithium and sodium and fluid balance. Lithium and sodium affect the fluid balance in the body. Therefore, patients who are taking lithium must maintain an adequate intake of fluids and salt. A decrease in the intake of either or both of these increases the potential for lithium retention, which will cause the serum level of lithium to rise. Alternatively, if the intake of sodium or fluids or both is increased, the amount of lithium excreted increases, causing a decrease in the serum level of lithium. Patients should follow their physician's advice if they are on a low-salt diet, take diuretics, change their intake of sodium or fluids, or perspire a lot as all these can affect the serum lithium levels.

Lithium toxicity can be fatal. This situation is progressive and can be detected early by monitoring for lithium's toxic effects and measuring serum blood levels. Some early indicators of toxic effects include the following (Long, 2003):

- Fainting
- Lethargy and sluggishness
- Slurred speech
- Nausea, vomiting, and diarrhea
- Hypotension, arrhythmias, pulse irregularities
- Thirst, dry mouth, bloated stomach
- Tremors, especially of the hands
- Ataxia
- Weight gain

The more pronounced signs include the following:

- Muscle fasciculations
- Seizures
- Change in consciousness
- Electrolyte imbalance
- Cardiac problems

No antidote is available for treating lithium toxicity. The drug is discontinued and the patient is treated symptomatically.

Side Effects

Lithium has common side effects seen in patients which can jeopardize their compliance with lithium therapy. These include the following (Long, 2003):

- Nausea
- Vomiting
- Diarrhea
- Excessive urination
- Abdominal cramping

- Hand tremors
- Muscle weakness, stiffness
- Fatigue, sluggishness
- Weight gain
- Metallic taste in the mouth

In addition, impairment in kidney or thyroid functioning, which is usually reversible, may occur with long-term use. Patients on long-term lithium therapy should have a complete physical examination every 6 months, including a check of kidney and thyroid functioning.

Contraindications

Patients should have a physical examination before lithium therapy is started. The drug should be used cautiously in patients who have the following:

- Cardiac problems
- Myasthenia gravis
- Organic brain syndrome
- Seizure disorders
- Parkinson's disease
- Pregnancy (also women who are lactating)
- Kidney problems
- Thyroid disorders

As with many potent medications, the potential benefits must be weighed against the potential risks. This list is not complete, and each patient's physical condition should be considered before treatment with lithium is begun.

Alternatives Medications to Lithium

Bipolar disorder is also treated with divalproex (Depakote®), which has been used as an anticonvulsant. It produces a rapid therapeutic response and serious complications with this medication are rare. It can cause sedation, weight gain, tremor and gastrointestinal problems. It has also been known to cause hepatic failure (Spratto & Woods, 2003).

Other anticonvulsants used as mood stabilizers are:

- Carbamazepine (Tegretol®, Carbatrol®): Side effects include sedation and gastrointestinal disturbances; rarely, a risk of bone marrow suppression and liver inflammation.
- Lamotrigine (Lamictal®): Side effects include serious rash; may cause dizziness, headaches, and difficulties with vision.
- Gabapentin (Neurontin®): Side effects include fatigue, sedation, and dizziness.
- Topiramate (Topamax®): Side effects include sedation, dizziness, and cogitative slowing, memory difficulties. Contraindicated with patients with kidney stones; does not cause weight gain (Spratto & Woods, 2003).

NURSING INTERVENTIONS

Patients who need a psychotropic medication have been experiencing some problem with their emotions, cognition, or behavior. As with communication and interpersonal skills, the administration of these medications requires knowledge and special consideration from the nurse.

The following interventions can be used for patients who are taking a psychotropic medication:

- Follow the health care facility protocol for administration of these medications.
- Review the patient's history for contraindications to the prescribed medications.
- Interview the patient to determine prescribed, over-the-counter, and illegal drugs they may be taking in order to determine potential drug interactions.
- Assess the patient for baseline physiological and behavioral data.
- Monitor the patient's vital signs, daily intake and output, and weight as appropriate.

- Administer the medication as prescribed to the right patient, in the correct does, by the correct route.
- Assess for potential side effects.
- Assess the drug tolerance, physical and psychological dependence (when appropriate).
- Assess for evidence of the medication's effectiveness in alleviating the target symptoms.
- Monitor patient's response to medication treatment.
- Review medication regimen with health care team.
- Educate patients about their medication regimen and about the lag time between starting their medication and their symptoms lessening.
- Instruct the patient to report adverse symptoms. For example, if a patient is prescribed on an antipsychotic drug they should notify you, or their physician, if they develop a sore throat, fever, malaise, unusual bleeding, or motor restlessness.
- Instruct patients experiencing drowsiness or dizziness as a result of their psychotropic medications not to operate dangerous machinery or participate in activities that require mental alertness.
- Instruct patients on lithium to maintain adequate intake of sodium.
- If patients have been taking a medication long term, instruct them to not stop taking it abruptly because it might produce withdrawal symptoms, such as nausea, vomiting, tachycardia, insomnia, and tremulousness.
- Instruct patients to use sunscreen and wear protective clothing when outdoors, as appropriate.
- Educate the patient's family or caregiver(s), as appropriate, about their medication regimen.
- Encourage patients to carry identification on them describing the medication(s) they are taking.
- Document administration of medications in the patient's record.

CASE STUDY

A 60-year-old woman was markedly depressed after cardiac surgery. Her physician prescribed a low dose of amitriptyline for her to take each night and described the medication as an antidepressant that would bring her relief.

The patient began taking the medication at home but found herself becoming more and more unhappy. She awakened each night at 2 a.m.; she had no appetite; and although she had been encouraged to take short walks, she found herself too tired. She began sobbing uncontrollably and felt internally agitated.

After only 4 days on the medication, she attempted to commit suicide by taking an overdose of sleeping pills and left a note that read, "I am such a failure, even the antidepressant couldn't cure me. I might as well end my life now and no longer be a burden to anyone." This patient surely would have benefited from the knowledge of how long it takes before an antidepressant results in symptomatic relief.

After being hospitalized for the suicide attempt, the patient recovered without any adverse effects. She continued her antidepressant medication under the close supervision of the nursing staff. They advised her that the optimal therapeutic level of the antidepressant she was taking was achieved in 3-4 weeks. Upon discharge from the hospital, she was to be visited by a home health psychiatric nurse and remained under the care of a psychiatrist.

SUMMARY

Patients are prescribed psychotropic medications to treat the symptoms related to their emotional problems and mental illnesses. Nurses are legally and ethically responsible for knowing the psychotropic medications their patients are prescribed, including the action, dosage, adverse effects, and potential drug interactions.

EXAM QUESTIONS

CHAPTER 14

Questions 82-89

82. _____ are classified as antipsychotic medications.
    a. Thorazine® and Clozaril®
    b. Mellaril® and Elavil®
    c. Elavil® and BuSpar®
    d. Valium® and Librium®

83. _____ are classified as anxiolytics medications.
    a. Clonazepam and Clozaril®
    b. Thorazine® and Diazepam
    c. Haldol® and Amobarbital
    d. Xanax® and Paxipam®

84. _____ are classified as antidepressants.
    a. Prozac®, Norpramin®
    b. Halcion®, Haldol®
    c. Desyrel®, Ambien®
    d. Elavil®, Mellaril®

85. Antipsychotic medications are used to treat
    a. toxic reactions and hallucinations.
    b. delusions and hallucinations.
    c. depression.
    d. extrapyramidal side effects.

86. Dystonia and drug-induced parkinsonism are examples of potential side effects of
    a. antipsychotics.
    b. anxiolytics.
    c. antidepressants.
    d. mood stabilizers.

87. When started on a tricyclic antidepressant, it generally takes ___________ of continuous use before beneficial results are seen.
    a. 12 hours
    b. 1 day
    c. 1 week
    d. 2-3 weeks

88. The nurse instructs the patient that addiction is a potential danger associated with use of
    a. some antipsychotics.
    b. Haldol®.
    c. lithium carbonate.
    d. some anxiolytics.

89. The nurse instructs the patient that a toxic serum level of lithium is
    a. 1.00 mEq/L.
    b. 1.25 mEq/L.
    c. 1.50 mEq/L.
    d. 2.50 mEq/L.

CHAPTER 15

ETHICAL AND LEGAL ISSUES IN PSYCHIATRIC NURSING

CHAPTER OBJECTIVE

After completing this chapter, the reader will be able to recognize ethical and legal concerns in the practice of nursing when dealing with patients having psychiatric and mental health problems.

LEARNING OBJECTIVES

After studying this chapter, the reader will be able to

1. recognize ethical principles related to nursing practice.
2. cite the provisions in the American Nurses Association (ANA) Code for Nurses, and the Standards of Practice for Psychiatric-Mental Health Nursing.
3. discuss current issues in the ethical and legal aspects of nursing practice.

OVERVIEW

Ethical and legal issues go hand in hand. All areas and specialties of nursing are affected by issues of ethics and matters pertaining to the legal aspects of health care. Ethics in nursing practice is concerned with doing good for patients while avoiding harm to them. Ethical issues are those involving decisions whereby a moral judgment comes into play. Legal issues in nursing practice are those matters that not only require a moral judgment but also are mandated by the justice system. In dealing with these issues, nurses are held accountable, and therefore punishable, by law.

ETHICAL ISSUES

Ethical Principles

Ethical principles are basic truths or laws that guide conduct and behavior and provide the framework for the practice of professional nursing.

The ethical principles most essential for nurses to understand to provide ethical nursing care are autonomy, non-maleficence, veracity, beneficence, justice, and fidelity.

- *Autonomy* (Advocacy): Autonomy is the respect for the person to make individual choices; that is, to self-determine. To give ethical nursing care, you must respect your patient's right to make health care decisions. Informed consent arises from the principles of autonomy and veracity.
- *Non-maleficence:* Non-maleficence means to do no harm or minimize harm. You must avoid causing harm and strive to protect patients from harm, and you do so by following acceptable standards of practice. Intentional harm is unacceptable in nursing. However, there may be risk of harm from an intervention that is intended to be helpful (e.g., pain medication given to relieve suffering could hasten death).

- *Veracity:* Veracity is truth telling. You are to always tell the truth and never lie or deceive patients. (It formerly was common not to tell patients what their diagnosis or prognosis was.) This principle also relates to the principle of autonomy because patients can only make the best health care decisions when given accurate information about their situation.
- *Beneficence:* Beneficence means doing the greatest good for patients. Their well-being is of sole importance. This must be balanced with risk of harm, especially, with the advanced technology in today's health care arena. You have an obligation to implement actions beneficial to the patients. For example, failing to turn a bedridden patient who complains of pain during such procedures may produce the short-term good of reduced discomfort. But it may also cause the harm of impaired skin integrity and musculoskeletal deformities.
- *Justice:* Justice is fairness, equitable use of resources, and equal access to health care. It is concerned with fair and equal treatment of all patients and equal access to health care for all people.
- *Fidelity:* Fidelity means faithfulness to the agreements and responsibilities undertaken. It means keeping your promises. It is the essence of a trusting relationship between nurses and patients. When you say, "I'll give you your medication at 1:00 p.m.," your patient hears it as a promise. It is your responsibility to keep your commitments to patients. If you are unable to, you must inform your patients and have an alternate plan (Thobaben, 2003).

Nurses are confronted with ethical dilemmas in all areas of nursing practice. To help solve an ethical dilemma, use the ethical decision-making process. Refer to Table 15-1: Ethical Decision-Making Process for suggested steps in making an ethical decision.

TABLE 15-1: ETHICAL DECISION-MAKING PROCESS
• Identify the problem (Determination and acknowledgment of the ethical conflict)
• Identify the ethical issues
• Define personal and professional moral positions and legal positions if applicable
• Identify value conflicts
• Identify all those involved in making the decision, and determine who should make the decision
• Identify each of the actions possible, and explore alternatives
• Selection and implementation of a course of action
• Evaluate results

CODE FOR NURSES

The ANA Code for Nurses (ANA, 2001) offers guidelines for nursing practice. The specific provisions of this code are as follows:

1. The nurse, in all professional relationships, practices with compassion and respect for the inherent dignity, worth, and uniqueness of every individual, unrestricted by considerations of social or economic status, personal attributes, or the nature of health problems.
2. The nurse's primary commitment is to the patient, whether an individual, family, group, or community.
3. The nurse promotes, advocates for, and strives to protect the health, safety, and rights of the patient.
4. The nurse is responsible and accountable for individual nursing practice and determines the appropriate delegation of tasks consistent with the nurse's obligation to provide optimum patient care.
5. The nurse owes the same duties to self as to others, including the responsibility to preserve

integrity and safety, to maintain competence, and to continue personal and professional growth.

6. The nurse participates in establishing, maintaining, and improving health care environments and conditions of employment conducive to the provision of quality health care and consistent with the values of the profession through individual and collective action.
7. The nurse participates in the advancement of the profession through contributions to practice, education, administration, and knowledge development.
8. The nurse collaborates with other health professionals and the public in promoting community, national, and international efforts to meet health care needs.
9. The profession of nursing, as represented by associations and their members, is responsible for articulating nursing values, for maintaining the integrity of the profession and its practice, and for shaping social policy (ANA, 2001).

STANDARDS OF PRACTICE FOR PSYCHIATRIC NURSES

The ANA also provides standards of practice for different specialty groups within the nursing profession, which describe standards of care that pertain to professional nursing activities. A partial listing of the ANA's Standards of Psychiatric-Mental Health Clinical Nursing Practice (2000) includes:

I. The psychiatric-mental health nurse collects patient health data.

II. The psychiatric-mental health nurse analyzes the assessment data in determining diagnoses.

III. The psychiatric-mental health nurse identifies expected outcomes individualized to the patient.

IV. The psychiatric-mental health nurse develops a plan of care that is negotiated among the patient, nurse, family, and health care team and prescribes evidence-based interventions to attain expected outcomes.

V. The psychiatric-mental health nurse implements the interventions identified in the plan of care.

VI. The psychiatric-mental health nurse uses counseling interventions to assist patients in improving or regaining their previous coping abilities, fostering mental health, and preventing mental illness and disability. This standard is concerned with specific psychiatric-mental health nurse interventions: milieu therapy (providing a therapeutic environment), self-care activities (fostering self-care), psychobiologic interventions (has knowledge of), health teaching, case management, health promoting and health maintenance, and psychotherapy.

VII. The psychiatric-mental health nurse evaluates the patient's progress in attaining expected outcomes (ANA, 2000; Stuart, 2002).

Nurses who work with psychiatric patients or deal with psychosocial issues in any health care setting follow many of these standards, and all nurses in any field should be guided by the ANA Code for Nurses.

LEGAL ISSUES

The legal aspects of health care delivery services provided by practitioners are guided by criminal law. All persons as members of society are also bound by criminal law. In addition, mental health laws give further guidance in situations that include persons who may be harmful to themselves, or others, or are judged unable to care for themselves because they are significantly disabled by virtue of having a mental illness.

Least Restrictive Alternative

The concept of least restrictive alternative stems from a legal decision made in the case of Rouse v. Cameron in 1966. It was ruled that the court could no longer order a patient to be "hospitalized" involuntarily if reasonable alternative treatment plans could be offered. If treatment is not a part of the involuntary hospitalization, the patient may participate in a therapeutic program through an outpatient clinic, day hospital, residential treatment center, or group home. Patients will benefit most from this arrangement if they have sufficient social, family, and community supports to use these means as an adjunct to individual or group and family counseling.

The state can insist on treating a patient. In the best interests of the mentally ill who cannot care for themselves, each state does have the right to provide sufficient care and treatment, but it must offer this in the least restrictive manner available.

This issue has ethical concerns as well as legal ramifications. Those who believe in absolute rights for all persons, despite handicaps or disabilities, take issue with the paternalistic power the government is exhibiting in the role of caretaker or surrogate parent to someone who is mentally ill.

Involuntary Hospitalization

The courts continue to determine the need for involuntary hospitalization for persons who are considered to be a danger to themselves or others or who are so incapacitated by their mental illness that they cannot care for themselves. The ethical questions continue and will thus keep the issue of individual liberty alive.

Whereas the concept of the least restrictive alternative is applied to degree and means of treatment, the involuntary hospitalization of someone pertains to a most basic right. The Constitution of the United States guarantees all persons the right to pursue liberty. When the court orders involuntary hospitalization of someone who has not committed a crime, it is depriving that person of his or her basic right to be free.

The alternative point of view focuses on the mentally ill person who is considered to pose a clear and present danger to himself or herself or others, someone who is suicidal or homicidal and refuses treatment. In these instances, the government has the right to hospitalize that person involuntarily on a temporary basis. Additionally, it is the responsibility of the state to maintain the welfare of the public and keep it free from potential harm as may sometimes be the case.

Procedures, which are similar from state to state, delineate the process of involuntary hospitalization as practiced in each jurisdiction. The rights of the mentally ill person are protected by the inclusion of the following:

- Notification of when and why a commitment procedure will be held.
- A specified amount of time, which may differ from state to state, for which someone may be held against his or her will pending a formal hearing (varies, but generally from 48-92 hr, and is authorized by a certified mental health provider without court approval).
- Representation by an attorney and access to this legal counsel in an unobstructed manner.
- Some clear and convincing proof of dangerousness or inability to function. (The Supreme Court ruled on this issue in 1979, in the case of Addington v. Texas.)

Involuntary hospitalization because of a court order is for a specified period. At the end of that period, the patient is entitled to an additional hearing (in some states known as a Probable Cause Review) if there is further need or disagreement on the need for continued hospitalization. Although general hospital nurses they are not involved in the process, nurses should be aware of their own state mandates.

Right to Refuse Treatment

The past 40 years have seen the increasing use of psychotropic medications in the treatment of the mentally ill. Although these medications may produce some remarkable and dramatic changes in a patient's aberrant behavior, they are not without their own side effects, and some patients may not want to take them.

This issue of a patient's right to refuse medication has posed controversies in some cases, such as with patients who are hospitalized involuntarily. The case of Rennie v. Klein (1983) addressed the right of an involuntary patient to refuse treatment. The court ruled "on the basis of the right to privacy that mentally ill patients in nonemergency situations could refuse treatment." In addition to the right to refuse psychotropic medications, the right to refuse treatment may pertain to the use of involuntary seclusion and mechanical restraint.

Informed Consent

Tied to the issue of the patient's right to refuse treatment is the issue of informed consent. To agree to or refuse treatment, the patient must be aware of what the proposed treatment includes the reasons for it, the possible dangers, and any alternatives available. The ethical principle of autonomy is the basis for informed consent.

Informed consent is an issue throughout the general hospital and in general nursing practice. Patients have the right to be informed of their diagnosis, the nature and purpose and prognosis or expected outcome of their treatment, and to be given information about alternative treatments.

Usually informed consent for operative and other invasive procedures falls in the domain of the physician. Review of the informed consent may at times fall to the nurse, and if the nurse thinks the patient does not adequately understand the procedure the nurse must notify the physician.

In addition to providing information about medical procedures nurses have a responsibility to inform patients about nursing procedures which might be performed.

Competency

Mental competency refers to a person's ability to think clearly, to display insight into their current situation, and to make sound judgments. A competent person should be given the opportunity to give informed consent about medical treatment. In most instances, persons who have reached age 18 are permitted to manage their own health in any manner that they desire.

Legally, someone is not considered incompetent until a court declares the person incompetent and appoints a guardian or conservator to act on his or her behalf as guardian of his or her person or estate or both.

Patients' Rights

When patients are institutionalized, their rights as patients are preserved according to the guidelines of the particular institution they are in. The rights of all patients in general hospitals are guided by the American Hospital Association's Patient's Bill of Rights (1992). This bill defines the following rights of patients:

- The patient has the right to considerate and respectful care.
- The patient has the right to and is encouraged to obtain from physicians and other direct caregivers relevant, current, and understandable information about diagnosis, treatment, and prognosis.
- The patient has the right to make decisions about the plan of care before and during the course of treatment and to refuse a recommended treatment or plan of care to the extent permitted by law and to be informed of the medical consequences of this action.
- The patient has the right to have an advance directive concerning treatment or designating a surrogate decision maker with the expectation

that the hospital will honor the intent of that directive to the extent permitted by law and hospital policy.

- The patient has the right to every consideration of privacy.
- The patient has the right to expect that all communications and records pertaining to his or her care will be treated as confidential by the hospital, except in cases such as suspected abuse and public health hazards, when reporting is permitted or required by law.
- The patient has a right to review the records pertaining to his or her medical care and to have the information explained or interpreted as necessary, except when restricted by law.
- The patient has the right to expect that, within its capacity and policies, a hospital will make an appropriate and reasonable response to the request of a patient for appropriate and medically indicated care and services.
- The patient has the right to ask about and be informed of the existence of business relationships among the hospital, educational institutions, other health care providers, or payers that may influence the patient's treatment and care.
- The patient has the right to consent to or decline to participate in proposed research studies or human experimentation that affect care and treatment or require direct involvement of patients and to have those studies fully explained before the patient gives consent.
- The patient has the right to expect reasonable continuity of care when appropriate and to be informed by physicians and other caregivers of available and realistic care options when hospital care is no longer appropriate.
- The patient has the right to be informed of hospital policies and practices that relate to patients' care, treatment, and responsibilities.

Confidentiality

Understanding the issues of confidentiality and privilege is imperative when providing therapeutic care to patients. Confidentiality is the legal and ethical responsibility to keep all information about patients private. You are not to divulge information about patients unless the person has authorized access to the information.

The Health Insurance Portability and Accountability Act of 1996

The Health Insurance Portability and Accountability Act of 1996 (HIPAA) provides patients with greater control over personal health care information. HIPAA took effect on April 14, 2003. The Department of Health and Human Services (HHS) developed new standards to provide patients with access to their medical records and more control over how their personal health information is used and disclosed.

The new privacy regulations include the following standards (USHHS, 2003):

- *Access To Medical Records*: Patients may and obtain copies of their medical records and can request corrections if they identify errors and mistakes.
- *Notice of Privacy Practices*: Physicians and other health care providers must provide notice to their patients of how they might use personal medical information.
- *Limits on Use of Personal Medical Information*: This sets limits on how health plans and covered providers may use individually identifiable health information.
- *Prohibition on Marketing*: This sets new restrictions and limits on the use of patient information for marketing purposes.
- *Confidential Communications*: Patients can request that their physicians, health plans, and other covered entities take reasonable steps to ensure that all communications with the patient are confidential (USHHS, 2003).

Duty to Warn

Relevant to working with the mentally ill is the 1976 decision in the case of Tarasoff v. Regents of the University of California. This case mandated that a health care professional has the duty to warn the intended victim when a patient threatens to harm another individual, therapists to warn the individual, the individual's family or friends, or the authorities. This duty takes precedence over the duty to protect client confidentiality (Biers, 2003).

Advance Directives

Advance Directives are the result of the Patient Self-Determination Act (PSDA) of 1990. An advance directive is a written document, completed when a person is competent, which allows patients to specify their health care preferences prior to a situation that leaves them incapable of indicating their treatment choices. State laws vary in the types of advance directives available, such as living wills and durable power of attorney for health care.

CASE STUDY

The Suicidal Patient

A 26-year-old woman, Ms. Jarrod, was brought by ambulance to the emergency department of a large medical center. A neighbor had found the patient moaning and lying on the floor her apartment just inside the door. The patient's left hand had been almost severed.

The patient, had a history of paranoid schizophrenia and depression. Although she was in shock and not communicative, it appeared to the neighbor and the ambulance attendants that she had cut her own wrist with a meat cleaver.

The ambulance attendants had carefully packed the partially severed hand in saline, wrapping it well and keeping it close to the patient's arm. She was admitted directly to the operating room, where a microsurgery team was quickly assembled to perform the procedure to reattach her hand that ultimately took 14 hr to complete.

After the surgery, the patient was taken to the recovery room, where she awoke in a few hours. Her vital signs were stabilizing and her left arm was elevated held up to an IV pole by a complicated pulley system of gauze wrap. The surgery was considered successful. The hand was fully reattached and within a few days it would be more apparent how much return of functioning could be expected.

The recovery room nurse knew that up to this point, Ms. Jarrod had not spoken with anyone. The nurse was concerned that on awakening the patient would still be suicidal. While the patient slept, the usual routine of one nurse for two patients seemed sufficient. Once the patient was awake, her nurse instituted the following psychosocial nursing care measures:

- *A mental status examination was performed when the patient was awake and alert.*
- *A lethality assessment was made of the patient's current suicidal ideation.*
- *Constant observation was initiated. A nursing aide would stay with the patient at all times. In order to be effective, this meant within arm's length and always within eye view. If the aide needed relief, direct switch of staff members was done; the patient was never left alone.*
- *A bedside search was done. Potentially dangerous objects were removed. The usual bedside treatment setup (e.g., instruments, wound cleanser) was removed after each use.*
- *The patient's family was notified. Her parents, who lived in another state, made plans to visit immediately.*
- *The patient's therapist, a clinical nurse specialist, was notified, as was the psychiatrist the patient had been seeing for medication therapy.*
- *Although Ms. Jarrod said that she did not feel suicidal, the severity of her initial attempt was*

so great that until her therapist arrived, it was thought best for the staff to maintain the one-to-one constant watch.

Ms. Jarrod was transferred to a surgical unit. The nurses there already had been apprised of the situation, one that can be uncomfortable for general hospital nurses. The patient's primary nurse on the surgical unit already was working out a plan that would follow the guidelines of the recovery room staff:

- *She was put in a private room next to the nurses' station and within eye view of it.*
- *Her room was assessed for potential danger.*
- *Sharp objects and cleaning agents were removed.*
- *Treatment materials were not kept at her bedside.*
- *Her chart was clearly marked: SUICIDE PRECAUTIONS.*
- *The stimuli in this busy surgical room was decreased as much as possible.*

Communications with the patient made it clear that she was psychotic and quite paranoid. Although she remained quiet, when asked directly she clearly described voices that she heard telling her "bad things" (i.e., " They told me to cut off my arm so I would be forgiven. The poisons needed a way to drain out.") When not communicating, she was observed to be apparently hallucinating; she was attentive to something and was seen talking animatedly to no one present.

Other interventions were:

- *She was under constant observation, with one-on-one nursing staff supervision in her room.*
- *Thirty min of each shift was spent sitting at her bedside encouraging her verbalization and to begin a trusting relationship with her.*
- *At least once each shift, she was asked about her suicidal ideation and an assessment was made of her mental status.*
- *The nurse was supportive and reassuring. When some new or painful procedure needed to be done, she tried to be there.*
- *Antipsychotic and antidepressant medications were started as ordered.*
- *A patient care conference with all the team members present was called to develop a care plan that all would consistently follow.*
- *She was observed swallowing her medications, so there would be no opportunity for her to cheek and save them up for a possible future overdose.*
- *Reality testing and reorientation were done.*

The primary nurse tried to monitor the severity of the patient's psychosis and to report the same, noting any changes from the previous day or days. She carefully documented the care plan and ensuing events in the patient's chart, making sure to put in specific things the patient had said so that all staff members would understand what was meant by hallucinations, paranoid ideation, and suicidal ideation.

After 8 days on the postsurgical unit, the patient's condition had stabilized enough so she could be transferred to a locked inpatient unit in the psychiatric clinic attached to the hospital. The primary nurse continued to visit every 2 or 3 days at the request of the psychiatric staff and the patient who had begun a trusting and rewarding relationship with her.

SUMMARY

The legal and ethical issues of nursing and those specifically pertaining to psychiatric nursing interrelate when a nurse is working with a patient at any health care facility who may be mentally ill. These areas of ethical and legal concern need to be examined carefully. When in doubt about nursing implications, nurses should consult with other members of the health care team and their own supervisors for guidelines. In professional nursing practice, it is important to maintain confidential relationships with patients and an awareness of current legal and ethical issues.

EXAM QUESTIONS

CHAPTER 15

Questions 90-95

90. Autonomy as an ethical principle means
    a. respect for the person to make individual choices.
    b. to do no harm or minimize harm.
    c. truth telling.
    d. doing the greatest good for patients.

91. The nurse maintains competence in nursing is a specific provision in the
    a. ANA's Code for Nurses.
    b. Patient's Bill of Rights.
    c. Professional Practice Guidelines.
    d. Standards of Practice for Psychiatric and Mental Health Nursing.

92. The following are two current ethical issues in psychiatric nursing
    a. involuntary hospitalization and right to life.
    b. least restrictive alternative and right to die.
    c. informed consent and right to vote.
    d. least restrictive alternative and involuntary hospitalization.

93. The legal concern addressed in the Tarasoff decision is
    a. informed consent versus right to life.
    b. competency versus commitment.
    c. duty to warn versus confidentiality.
    d. privilege versus confidentiality.

94. A psychiatric patient refuses to take any medication. She states she does not need it. She is actively hallucinating and gravely disabled. If this response continues, you should recommend that she
    a. hide her medication in her food.
    b. refuse medication based on her right to refuse treatment.
    c. take her medication against her will.
    d. start conservatorship proceedings.

95. The Health Insurance Portability and Accountability Act of 1996 sets standards to
    a. increase reimbursement for physicians.
    b. give patient's right to refuse treatment.
    c. give more control to patients over how their personal health information is used and disclosed.
    d. allow health insurance companies more flexibility in funding.

CHAPTER 16

NURSING MANAGEMENT OF PATIENTS WITH SLEEP DISORDERS

CHAPTER OBJECTIVE

After completing this chapter, the reader will be able to recognize the signs and symptoms of sleep disorders and be able to apply sound principles of nursing care to patients experiencing sleep disorders.

LEARNING OBJECTIVES

After studying this chapter, the reader will be able to

1. describe the various types of *DSM-IV-TR* sleep disorders.
2. list the NANDA nursing and *DSM-IV-TR* diagnoses pertinent to sleep disorders.
3. identify nursing interventions that may be effective with patients experiencing sleep disorders.

OVERVIEW

Sleep is necessary for survival. According to the National Institute of Neurological Disorders and Stroke (NINDS, 2003), most adults need 7-8 hr of sleep per night to feel alert and not have the urge to nap; although some may need as few as 5 hr or as many as 10 hr of sleep each day. The amount of sleep each person needs depends on many factors, including age and individual life-style. Infants generally require about 16 hr a day, while teenagers need about 9 hr on average (NINDS, 2003).

During sleep, a person usually passes rapid eye movement through five phases of sleep: stages 1, 2, 3, 4, and (REM) sleep, and then the cycle starts over again with stage 1 (NINDS, 2003).

At least 40 million Americans suffer from chronic, long-term sleep disorders each year, and an additional 20 million experience occasional sleeping problems (NINDS, 2003).

The most common sleep disorders include insomnia, sleep apnea, restless-legs syndrome, and narcolepsy, which can be managed effectively once they are correctly diagnosed (NINDS, 2003). It is important to diagnose and treat sleep disorders and the underlying medical or psychological problems that may be associated with them.

TYPES OF SLEEP DISORDERS

According to the American Psychiatric Association, sleep disorders are classified into the following four categories based on presumed etiology (*DSM-IV-TR*, 2000):

- *Primary Sleep Disorder*: The complaint of sleep disturbance arises from endogenous abnormalities in sleep-wake generating or timing mechanisms, often complicated by conditioning factors.
- *Sleep Disorder Related to an Another Mental Disorder*: The complaint of sleep disturbance

that is the result of a diagnosable mental disorder (often mood disorder or anxiety disorders). The pathophysiological mechanisms responsible for the mental disorder also affect sleep-wake regulation.

- *Sleep Disorder Due to a General Medical Condition*: The complaint of sleep disturbance results from direct physiological effects of a general medical condition on the sleep-wake system.
- *Substance-Induced Sleep Disorder*: The complaint of sleep disturbance is from the concurrent use, or recent discontinuation use, of a substance (including medications).

Primary Sleep Disorders

Primary Sleep Disorders are subdivided into two categories: Dyssomnias (characterized by abnormalities in the amount, quality or timing of sleep), and Parasomnias (characterized by abnormal behavioral or physiological events occurring in association with sleep, specific sleep stages or the sleep-wake cycle (*DSM-IV-TR*, 2000).

Dyssomnias include primary insomnia, primary hypersomnia, narcolepsy, breathing-related disorder, circadian rhythm sleep disorder, and dyssomnia not otherwise specified.

Parasomnias are disorders associated with sleep stages and include nightmare disorder, sleep terror disorder, sleepwalking disorder, and parasomnia not otherwise specified.

DYSSOMNIA DISORDERS

Primary Insomnia

Primary insomnia is a sleep disturbance that occurs for at least 1 month during which the patient has a complaint of difficulty initiating or maintaining sleep or has nonrestorative sleep. It causes clinically significant distress or impairment in social, occupational, or other areas of functioning (*DSM-IV-TR*, 2000).

Characteristics include the following:

- Difficulty falling asleep
- Waking up frequently during the night
- Difficulty returning to sleep
- Waking up too early in the morning
- Unrefreshing sleep

Primary Hypersomnia

Primary hypersomnia is excessive sleepiness that is either prolonged sleep episodes or daytime sleep episodes occurring almost daily, which last for at least a month. The sleep episodes last for 8-12 hr, and are often followed by difficulty awakening in the morning. The patient's daytime naps are generally long and are unrefreshing (*DSM-IV-TR*, 2000). It causes clinically significant distress or impairment in social, occupational, or other areas of functioning. Often patients have symptoms of depression, and are at risk for substance-related disorders, particularly, use of stimulants (*DSM-IV-TR*, 2000).

Narcolepsy

Narcolepsy is a chronic disabling neurological disorder of sleep regulation with no known cause. It's essential features are irresistible attacks of refreshing sleep that occur daily over at least 3 months, cataplexy, and recurrent intrusions of elements of REM sleep into the transition between sleep and wakefulness (*DSM-IV-TR*, 2000).

Narcolepsy occurs in men and women at any age, although its symptoms are usually first noticed in teenagers or young adults. There is no cure for narcolepsy. Patients are often treated with stimulants and antidepressants to help control the symptoms. They are often encouraged to nap at certain times of the day to help reduce their excessive daytime sleepiness (NINDS, 2003, 2001).

Patients may experience some or all of the following symptoms:

- Drowsiness persisting for prolonged periods.

- Excessive and overwhelming daytime sleepiness, even after adequate nighttime sleep.
- Drowsiness or falling asleep, often at inappropriate times and places, such as at dinner, or while talking, driving, or working.
- Daytime sleep attacks, often repeated, occurring with or without warning which may be irresistible.
- Nighttime sleep fragmented with frequent awakenings.
- Cataplexy: brief episodes of sudden bilateral loss of muscle tone, (ranging from slight weakness, such as limpness at the neck or knees, sagging facial muscles, or inability to speak clearly, to complete body collapse most often associated with intense emotion, such as anger or fear. It may last from a few seconds to several minutes, and the person remains conscious throughout the episode.
- Sleep paralysis: temporary inability to talk or move when falling asleep or waking up, which may last from a few seconds to minutes.
- Hypnagogic hallucinations: vivid, often frightening, dream-like experiences that occur at the beginning or end of sleep episodes (*DSM-IV-TR*, 2000; NINDS, 2003, 2001).

Breathing-Related Disorder

The essential feature of breathing-related disorder is sleep disruption leading to excessive sleepiness or, less commonly, to insomnia that is judged to be due to abnormalities of ventilation during obstructive or central sleep apnea syndrome or central alveolar hypoventilation syndrome (*DSM-IV-TR*, 2000).

The most common form of breathing-related sleep disorder is obstructive sleep apnea syndrome. It is characterized by loud snores, or brief gasps that alternate with episodes of silence that usually last 20-30 seconds.

Sleep apnea is a serious, potentially life-threatening condition (*DSM-IV-TR*, 2000). It occurs when air cannot flow into or out of the person's nose or mouth although efforts to breathe continue (*DSM-IV-TR*, 2000).

Central sleep apnea syndrome, which is less common, occurs when the brain fails to send the appropriate signals to the breathing muscles to initiate respirations; it is characterized by episodic cessation of ventilation during sleep without airway obstruction (*DSM-IV-TR*, 2000).

Central alveolar hypoventilation syndrome results in abnormally low arterial oxygen levels further worsened by sleep due to impairment in ventilatory control (*DSM-IV-TR*, 2000).

The consequences of these disorders range from annoying to life-threatening. They include:

- Depression
- Irritability
- Sexual dysfunction
- Learning and memory difficulties
- Falling asleep while at work, on the phone, or driving
- Contributing to high blood pressure
- Risk for heart attack and stroke

Circadian Rhythm Sleep Disorder

According to the *DSM-IV-TR*, circadian rhythm sleep disorder is a persistent or recurrent pattern of sleep disruption leading to excessive sleepiness or insomnia that is due to a mismatch between the sleep-wake schedule required by a person's environment and their circadian sleep-wake pattern.

The subtypes include jet lag, shift work, and delayed sleep phase type which is characterized by a delay of circadian rhythms, including the sleep-wake cycle, relative to the demands of society. A person cannot fall asleep or awaken at a desired earlier time (*DSM-IV-TR,* 2000).

Dyssomnias Not Otherwise Specified

This category is for insomnias, hypersomnias, or circadian rhythm disturbances that do not meet criteria for specific dyssomnia (*DSM-IV-TR*, 2000). They include:

- Environmental factors, such as noise, light, frequent interruptions.
- Ongoing sleep deprivation.
- Restless-legs syndrome (RLS), including
  - Unpleasant sensations in the legs (one or both), and sometimes the arms as well.
  - Described as creeping, crawling, tingling, pulling, or painful.
  - Usually occurs in the calf area but may be felt anywhere from the thigh to the ankle.
  - Occurs when the person lies down or sits for prolonged periods of time, such as at a desk, riding in a car, or watching a movie.
  - Produces an irresistible urge to move the legs when the sensations occur.
  - Worsens during periods of relaxation and decreased activity.
  - Follows a set daily cycle, with evening and night hours being more troublesome for RLS sufferers than morning hours.
  - Makes it difficult to relax and fall asleep because of a strong urge to walk or do other activities to relieve unpleasant sensations.
  - Best sleep is obtained toward the end of the night or during the morning hours.
  - Causes an overall difficulty falling asleep or staying asleep (*DSM-IV-TR*, 2000).

Parasomnia Disorders

Parasomnia disorders are associated with sleep stages and include nightmare disorder, sleep terror disorder, sleepwalking disorder and parasomnia not otherwise specified. They are characterized by abnormal behavioral or physiological events occurring with sleep, specific sleep stages, or sleep-wake transitions (*DSM-IV-TR,* 2000).

- *Nightmare Disorder:* Repeated awakenings with detailed recall of extended and extremely frightening dreams, usually a threat to survival, security or self-esteem (*DSM-IV-TR*, 2000).
- *Sleep Terror Disorder:* Repeated occurrence of sleep terrors — abrupt awakenings from sleep usually beginning with a panicky scream or cry (*DSM-IV-TR,* 2000).
- *Sleepwalking Disorder:* Repeated episodes of rising from the bed during sleep. The person is blank, has a staring face, and is relatively unresponsive to efforts to communicate with him/her. Can be awakened with great difficulty. Person has amnesia for the episode (*DSM-IV-TR*, 2000).

TREATMENT MODALITIES

To make a diagnosis of insomnia, a patient will need a complete physical and psychiatric examination to rule out medical or psychiatric conditions. The nurse may be involved in data collection. You should observe the patient for symptoms of sleep deprivation, such as dark circles under eyes, dozing, yawning, irritability, and impatience.

Interview the patient to obtain their sleeping pattern, family history of sleep disorders, current medications, and substance use.

The patient may be referred for formal sleep studies. Several tests are available for evaluating a person, such as the following (MEDLINEplus, 2003):

- *Polysomnography*: a test that monitors a variety of body functions during sleep, such as the electrical activity of the brain, eye movement, muscle activity, heart rate, respiratory effort, airflow, and blood oxygen levels.
- *The Multiple Sleep Latency Test (MSLT)*: measures the speed of falling asleep.

The most common pharmacologic interventions for acute primary insomnia are hypnotics.

These include benzodiazepines, such as temazepam (Restoril®) and nonbenzodiazepines, such as zolpidem (Ambien®).

In mild cases of RLS, activities such as walking, stretching, knee bends, a hot bath, massaging the legs, using a heating pad or ice pack, and eliminating caffeine may help to alleviate symptoms.

To correct breathing-related sleep disorders, surgery may be necessary to

- increase the size of the airway.
- remove adenoids and tonsils (especially in children), nasal polyps or other growths.
- remove excess tissue at the back of the throat, such as tonsils, uvula, and part of the soft palate, by performing an uvulopalatopharyngoplasty (UPPP).
- remove other tissue in the airway to correct structural deformities (Flagg, 2001).

If sleep difficulties are a result of mood or anxiety disorders, antidepressants are prescribed. If the patient has an underlying medical condition, such as sleep apnea, normal sleeping patterns should return once the condition is correct. Nonpharmacologic interventions, such as sleep hygiene, also help to establish normal sleep patterns.

DSM-IV-TR DIAGNOSES

The sleep disorder diagnoses that may be related to sleep disorders are

Primary Sleep Disorders

Dyssomnias

- Primary insomnia
- Primary hypersomnia
- Narcolepsy
- Breathing-related sleep disorder
- Circadian rhythm sleep disorder
- Dyssomnias not otherwise specified

Parasomnias

- Nightmare disorder (formerly dream anxiety disorder)
- Sleep terror disorder
- Sleepwalking disorder
- Parasomnia not otherwise specified

Sleep Disorder Due to a General Medical Condition

- Insomnia related to another mental disorder
- Hypersomnia related to another mental disorder
- Sleep disorder related to another mental disorder
- Substance-induced sleep disorder

NANDA NURSING DIAGNOSES

The NANDA nursing diagnoses that are related to sleep disorders indclude

- Anxiety
- Ineffective coping
- Fatigue
- Readiness for enhanced sleep
- Sleep deprivation
- Disturbed sleep pattern

NURSING INTERVENTIONS

- **Intervention**: Administer sleeping medications to patients as ordered. Assess its effectiveness and for side effects.

  Rationale: Sleeping medication can be effective in the treatment of sleep disturbances. Patients need to be assessed to determine if their medication was effective or if they experienced any side effects from it.
- **Intervention**: Instruct patients to take sleeping medication appropriately, such as:
  - Taking prescribed sleeping pill as ordered,

1 hr before bedtime to feel drowsy when going to sleep, and at least 10 hr before getting up to avoid daytime drowsiness.

- Not taking another person's sleeping pill, or over-the-counter sleeping pill without their doctor's knowledge.
- Encouraging use of sleep medication for short-term only.

Rationale: Sleeping medications are most effective when taken appropriately, and for the length of time ordered by the patient's physician.

- **Intervention**: Assist patients in identifying behaviors that may worsen their insomnia and offering ways to eliminate or reduce theses behaviors, such as:
  - Avoiding daytime napping.
  - Avoiding worrying before going to bed.
  - Avoiding foods and substances that interfere with sleep.

  Rationale: Helping patients understand what behaviors worsen their insomnia and ways to reduce these behaviors can help them eliminate or reduce their sleep disturbances.

- **Intervention**: Encourage patients to practice good sleep hygiene practices, such as:
  - Having a winding down period before going to bed.
  - Doing relaxation exercises before going to bed.
  - Developing a bedtime ritual.

  Rationale: Good hygiene practices can help patients eliminate or reduce their sleep disturbances (Table 16-1).

- **Intervention**: Instruct obese patient in nutritional counseling.

  Rationale: Obesity can result in daytime fatigue or sleep apnea.

SUMMARY

There are many types of sleep disorders. Both pharmacologic and nonpharmacologic interventions are available to help patients with sleep disorders. Instructing patients in good sleep hygiene practices can help them reduce sleep disturbances. Transient insomnia, such as occurs when a patient is hospitalized, may not require treatment since the episode may last only few days, and the patient's biological clock will go back to normal after discharge.

TABLE 16-1: SLEEP HYGIENE PRACTICES

Sleep Habits	Bedroom	Lifestyle
Go to bed at the same time each day.	Keep the temperature comfortable.	Get regular exercise each day, preferably in the morning includes stretching and aerobic exercise.
Get up from bed at the same time each day.	Keep room dark enough to facilitate sleep.	Get regular exposure to outdoor or bright lights, especially in the late afternoon.
Use your bed only for sleep and sex.	Keep the room quiet when sleeping.	Do not engage in stimulating activity just before bed, such as playing a competitive game, watching an exciting movie or program on television, or having an important discussion with significant other.
If you lay in bed awake for more than 20-30 min, get up, go to a different room (or different part of the bedroom); Do this as many times during the night as needed.	Remove the clock from bedroom or turn the clock so it is not visible.	Relax just before going to sleep by doing muscle relaxation, imagery, massage, warm bath, non-excitable reading, or watching television (but not in bed).
Do not command yourself to go to sleep. This only makes your mind and body more alert.		Do not use alcohol to help you sleep.
Do not read or watch television in bed.		Do not have caffeine in the evening (coffee, teas, chocolate, sodas).
Do not take daytime naps.		Do not go to bed too hungry or too full. Take diuretics early in the day. Empty bladder before going to sleep.
Keep your feet and hands warm. Wear warm socks and/or mittens or gloves to bed.		Avoid nicotine.

EXAM QUESTIONS

CHAPTER 16

Questions 96-100

96. A sleep disorder that is due to a general medical condition

    a. involves excessive sleepiness.
    b. involves unrefreshing sleep.
    c. results from direct physiological effects of a general medical condition on the sleep-wake system.
    d. can be seen in narcolepsy.

97. Dyssomnia sleep disorders include

    a. primary hypersomnia, sleep terror disorder.
    b. Narcolepsy, primary insomnia.
    c. Breathing-related disorder, sleepwalking disorder.
    d. Circadian rhythm, nightmare disorder.

98. Parasomnias sleep disorders include

    a. Sleepwalking disorder, sleep terror disorder.
    b. Narcolepsy, sleep apnea.
    c. Primary insomnia, primary hypersomnia.
    d. Circadian rhythm, night terrors.

99. A patient was prescribed zolpidem (Ambien) for a sleep disorder. He expressed concern about becoming addicted. Your best response is

    a. "The drug is highly addictive."
    b. "Don't worry the medication is not addictive."
    c. "I would advise you not to take it."
    d. "I understand your concerns, but it is only prescribed for 2 weeks."

100. An example of a poor sleep hygiene practice is

    a. keeping the bedroom dark enough to sleep.
    b. removing the clock from bedroom.
    c. not taking daytime naps.
    d. watching television in bed.

This concludes the final examination. An answer key will be sent with your certificate so that you can determine which of your answers were correct and incorrect.

RESOURCES

The American Academy of Child and Adolescent Psychiatry
3615 Wisconsin Ave., N.W.,
Washington, DC 20016-3007
202-966-7300
Fax: 202-966-2891
http://www.aacap.org/

Anxiety Disorders Association of America
8730 Georgia Avenue, Suite 600
Silver Springs, MD 20910
240-485-1001
Fax: 240-485-1035
http://www.adaa.org/

American Foundation for Suicide Prevention
120 Wall Street, 22nd Floor
New York, NY 10005
888-333-AFSP/212-363-3500
Fax: 212-363-6237
http://www.afsp.org/

American Psychiatric Association
1000 Wilson Boulevard, Suite 1825
Arlington, VA 22209-3901
703-907-7300
http://www.psych.org/

American Psychiatric Nurses Association
1555 Wilson Blvd., Suite 515
Arlington, VA 22209
703-243-2443
Fax: 703-243-3390
http://www.apna.org/

American Psychological Association
750 First Street, NE
Washington, DC 20002-4242
800-374-2721; 202-336-5510
TDD/TTY: 202-336-6123
http://www.apa.org/

American Psychological Society
1010 Vermont Avenue NW, Suite 1100
Washington, DC 20005-4907
202-783-2077
Fax: 202-783-2083
http://www.psychologicalscience.org/

Depression and Related Affective Disorders Association (DRADA)
2330 West Joppa Rd., Suite 100
Lutherville, MD 21093
410-583-2919
http://www.drada.org/

Eating Disorder Referral and Information Center
http://www.edreferral.com/

International Society of Psychiatric-Mental Health Nurses
http://www.ispn-psych.org/

Internet Mental Health: Disorders
http://www.mentalhealth.com/p20-grp.html

National Foundation For Depressive Illness, Inc.
P.O. Box 2257
New York, NY 10116
800-239-1265
http://www.depression.org/

The National Institute for Occupational Safety and Health (NIOSH)
Hubert H. Humphrey Bldg.
200 Independence Ave., SW, Room 715H
Washington, DC 20201
202-401-0721
http://www.cdc.gov/niosh/homepage.html

National Institute of Mental Health (NIMH)
Office of Communications
6001 Executive Boulevard, Room 8184
MSC 9663
Bethesda, MD 20892-9663
301-443-4513 or
1-866-615-NIMH (6464), toll-free
TTY: 301-443-8431; Fax: 301-443-4279
http://www.nimh.nih.gov

National Institute on Drug Abuse
National Institutes of Health
6001 Executive Boulevard, Room 5213
Bethesda, MD 20892-9561
301-443-1124
http://www.drugabuse.gov/

National Sleep Foundation
http://www.sleepfoundation.org/

Sleepnet.com™
http://www.sleepnet.com/

GLOSSARY

abuse: The continued use of substances (alcohol and other drugs) over a prolonged period of time even after problems occurs.

acuity: Intensity of illness stated as high acuity or low acuity; may refer to an individual's illness, or to the state of many patients within the milieu (i.e., a milieu with high acuity).

affect: The facial expression and body language that reflect or indicate an emotion.

akathisia: Motor restlessness as caused by the side effect of antipsychotic medications (major tranquilizers); often described by patients as an inability to sit still or to keep one's legs still; may be mistakenly assessed as anxiety or insomnia, because akathisia prevents lying still long enough to fall asleep.

alcoholism: A disorder characterized by out-of-control consumption of alcohol, resulting in biological, social, and vocational functional impairment.

amnestic disorder: A disorder characterized by severe impairment of both short- and long-term memory; usually with organic cause; may be psychogenic amnesia after stressful or conflictual events.

anhedonia: An impairment in the ability to experience pleasure; often accompanies depression.

anorexia: A loss of, or decrease in, appetite.

anorexia nervosa: An eating disorder in which the person affected is severely preoccupied with food, dieting, and body image; characterized by failure to maintain normal body weight while misperceiving one's body as "fat"; using laxatives, diuretics, and self-induced vomiting to lose weight; may be so severe as to lead to death.

anticholinergic side effects: A group of side effects that may occur with antipsychotic and antidepressant medications; includes dry mouth, constipation, blurred vision, urinary retention, mydriasis; more severe anticholinergic side effects may include agitation, confusion, hallucinations, and seizures.

antidepressants: Medications with a primary indication for the relief of depression; major categories of antidepressants include the tricyclic antidepressants (TCAs), the monoamine oxidase inhibitors (MAOIs), the selective serotonin reuptake inhibitors (SSRIs), and the second-generation antidepressants.

antipsychotics: Class of medications used for the alleviation of impaired thought processes (e.g., hallucinations, delusions) and/or a state of agitation; also referred to as major tranquilizers or neuroleptics.

anxiety: An unpleasant feeling of dread and apprehension. An emotional state, which may be a disorder in itself, a component of another emotional disorder (e.g., depression may be accompanied by anxiety), or an indication of a physical disorder (e.g., may accompany hypertension), characterized by internal restlessness, nervousness, and an inability to relax; may be of variable degrees of intensity; often rated on a scale of 1 to 4+, with 4+ being the most intense level of anxiety.

anxiety disorders: A group of disorders characterized primarily by anxiety; includes panic disorder, obsessive-compulsive disorder, generalized anxiety disorder, phobic disorders, and post-traumatic stress disorder.

anxiolytics: A class of medications used for the alleviation of signs and symptoms of anxiety or for the treatment of anxiety disorders; benzodiazepines fall within this class of medications.

benzodiazepines: A class of antianxiety medications with the intended effect of relief of anxiety; intended for short-term use, because long-term use may lead to psychological and physiological dependence and require medically monitored withdrawal; some medications in this class are also intended for use with alcohol withdrawal, insomnia, muscle relaxation, and/or treatment of panic disorders.

bipolar disorder: A major mental illness characterized by episodes of mania and depression; usually diagnosed when the affected person is in his or her 20s; frequency of episodes of mania or depression vary from patient to patient; treatment of choice is with mood-stabilizing medications, such as lithium carbonate.

borderline personality disorder: A personality disorder; may be seen with severe impairment in interpersonal relatedness and vocational functioning; characterized by emotional lability, reckless impulsiveness, inability to modulate anger, chronic feelings of emptiness or boredom, ineffective coping abilities, and recurrent suicidal thoughts or behaviors.

bulimia nervosa: An eating disorder characterized by uncontrolled eating of excessive amounts of food, which is often followed by feelings of guilt, self-hate, or depression; often accompanied by the use of laxatives or self-induced vomiting to counter the binge eating.

butyrophenones: Chemical class of antipsychotic medications; includes haloperidol.

cataplexy: brief episodes of sudden bilateral loss of muscle tone, which is most often associated with intense emotion.

cognitive abilities: A person's abilities of thinking, including the ability to reason, to make inferences, and to understand.

command hallucination: An auditory hallucination (see hallucinations) in which one or more voices instruct the affected person to act in a certain way; often a command that is dangerous to the person (e.g., jump off a bridge, walk in front of a car); the person who experiences the commands does not perceive any control over his or her response to them.

competency: Mental competency; refers to a person's ability to think clearly, to display insight into the current situation, and to make sound judgments; in a legal sense, a person is assumed to be competent unless deemed incompetent by a court of law.

concrete thinking: A lack of abstract thinking, seeing only the "night and day" of a situation, without the ability to go beyond to see the implied meaning, or more abstract meaning; making literal versus figurative interpretations of words or phrases.

coping ability: The skill or ability to manage the various challenges that occur as a regular part of a person's life; may be assessed for a person or for a family unit.

cyclothymic disorder: A mild form of bipolar affective illness (see bipolar affective illness).

delirium: A disordered mental status characterized by confusion, agitation, and hallucinations; has various physical or mental causes.

delirium tremens: A disordered mental state, or delirium, that occurs during withdrawal from alcohol; characterized by tremors, confusion, agitation, hallucinations, apprehension, and elevated vital signs; can lead to a medical emergency if not treated aggressively and in a timely manner.

delusion: A false belief as a manifestation of a thought disorder; may be of various types, including persecutory, religious, grandiose, somatic, bizarre, nihilistic, and self-deprecatory.

dementia: A progressive deterioration of the brain, of an organic nature; more than 50% of patients who have dementia have Alzheimer's disease; multi-infarct dementia and HIV dementia are other leading types; may cause variable degrees of impairment.

dependence: A cluster of cognitive, behavioral, and physiological symptoms indicating that the individual continues use of the substance despite significant substance-related problems.

depressive disorder: Referred to as major depression; may be a single episode or a recurring illness; often characterized by vegetative signs and symptoms (loss of appetite, insomnia or hypersomnia, decreased ability to concentrate, decreased libido), hopelessness or helplessness, sadness, anhedonia, agitation, withdrawal, negativity, and suicidal ideations and behaviors.

dihydroindolones: A class of antipsychotic medications; includes molindone.

diphenylbutylpiperidines: A class of antipsychotic medications; includes pimozide.

DSM-IV-TR: Acronym for the 2000 edition of *Diagnostic and Statistical Manual of Mental Disorders* published by the American Psychiatric Association; describes the various mental disorders and specific criteria needed to make a definitive diagnosis.

duty to warn: A group of statutes related to professional responsibilities to warn intended victims of a patient's statements of intent to harm; the most famous comes from the Tarasoff v. Regents of University of California case.

dyskinesias: Movement disorders characterized by difficulty of movement or involuntary movement.

dysthymic disorder: A mood disorder similar to depression, with chronic versus episodic signs and symptoms and general, overall unhappiness; often results in impairments in interpersonal and vocational functioning.

echolalia: Behavior in which the person affected automatically repeats what is said to him or her; may be present with a psychotic disorder.

extrapyramidal side effects: A group of side effects of the antipsychotics (major tranquilizers); more common with the higher potency ones; includes akathisia, pseudoparkinsonism, acute dystonic reactions, and tardive dyskinesia; named for the area of the brain involved.

fear: An unpleasant feeling caused by the realization and recognition that some event, occurrence, or other detectable source in the environment may bring harm.

flight of ideas: An alteration in thought processes characterized by the jumping from one idea to another unrelated idea, usually in rapid succession; often accompanies the manic phase of bipolar affective disorder.

grandiosity: An alteration in thought processes in which the affected person has delusional beliefs that he or she is of great importance or has superhuman abilities (e.g., the person may believe that he or she holds the key to world peace, or that he or she can fly like the birds).

hallucination: A sensory perception that occurs without external stimulation of the relevant sensory organ.

histrionic personality disorder: A personality disorder characterized by a constant need for approval, an exaggerated expression of emotion, a discomfort with not being the center of attention, and self-centeredness.

hypnagogic hallucinations: vivid, often frightening, dream-like experiences that occur at the beginning or end of sleep episodes.

hyper-religiosity: An abnormally high focus on religious ideas and beliefs; as a component of an emotional illness, often of a delusional nature.

hypersexuality: An abnormally high libido and focus on sexual thoughts as may accompany some psychiatric illnesses (e.g., the manic phase of bipolar disorder).

inappropriate affect: Facial expression or body language that is incongruent with the content of thought, mood, or emotion expressed.

insight: Awareness of one's situation and the factors affecting the situation; a lack of insight may accompany emotional disorders and compromise a person's ability to make appropriate decisions and use good, sound judgment.

lethargy: A psychobiological state in which the affected person has little energy, little interest or desires to mobilize his or her energies; sluggishness.

lithium carbonate: A mood-stabilizing medication.

looseness of association: An alteration in thought processes in which the affected person's speech reflects a lack of organized, sensible connectedness between subjects; for example, talks of feeling blue then jumps to the subject of the blue sky.

major depressive episode: Episodes of major depression that occurs more than once; may recur one time or several times over many years.

manic episode: See bipolar disorder.

manipulate: To get one's needs met indirectly, often at the expense of others, and often when a more direct expression of one's needs would be unsuccessful in achieving the desired result.

mental status examination: A comprehensive examination of a person's emotional state and thinking processes at a given point of time; when used in making a diagnosis of a psychiatric illness, the equivalent of a physical examination in making a physical diagnosis.

monoamine oxidase inhibitors (MAOIs): A class of antidepressant medications that works by inhibiting monoamine oxidase in the synaptic cleft; includes Nardil, Parnate, Marplan; patients taking these medications must follow a strict diet (no foods containing the amino acid tyramine) and should check with their physician before taking any over-the-counter medications; failure to follow the diet and medication restrictions could result in a hypertensive crisis.

mood: A person's emotion that colors his or her perception of the world and people around him or her.

mutism: Voicelessness with an emotional cause rather than a physical one.

neuroleptics: Medications that affect the brain and central nervous system.

noncompliance: Failure to follow the prescribed treatment regimen.

obsessive-compulsive disorder: A psychiatric disorder characterized by recurrent obsessional thinking and recurrent compulsive behaviors severe enough to interfere with normal interpersonal and vocational functioning.

organic anxiety disorder: An organic disorder characterized by recurrent panic attacks or by generalized anxiety.

organic delusional disorder: An organic disorder characterized by alteration in thought processes in which the person affected has false beliefs (see delusions); most often caused by use of drugs such as amphetamines, cannabis, and hallucinogens.

organic hallucinosis: An organic disorder characterized by alteration in thought processes in which the person affected has hallucinations; most often caused by chronic alcohol or drug abuse.

organic mood disorder: An organic disorder characterized by mood disturbances, either of depression or mania.

organic personality syndrome: An organic disorder characterized by marked changes in a person's personality; most often caused by head trauma or brain injury.

orthostatic hypotension: A sudden drop in blood pressure that occurs when a person changes position (e.g., changes from lying down to sitting or standing); often a side effect of use of some of the psychotropic medications.

panic: An episode of severe anxiety in which the person affected experiences fearfulness, apprehension, foreboding, diaphoresis, elevated vital signs, and changes in psychomotor activity along with the perception that if relief is not promptly obtained, the person will experience an unfortunate fate (such as, "going crazy" or "dying"); may be a single episode or recurring episodes.

phenothiazines: A major class of antipsychotic medications; includes aliphatics, piperidines, and piperazines.

piperidines: A subclass of the phenothiazines; includes thioridazine and mesoridazine.

piperazines: A subclass of the phenothiazines; includes fluphenazine, trifluoperazine, and perphenazine.

psychiatric: Pertaining to a person's emotional state and thought functioning.

psychomotor retardation: A dramatic decrease in a person's physical activity, as may accompany severe depression.

psychosis: A disordered state of thinking, often characterized by hallucinations or delusions; has a variety of causes; may be acute or an ongoing part of a persistent mental disorder.

psychosocial: Pertaining to those aspects of a person that are of psychological or social origins.

psychopharmacological: Pertaining to medications that have intended effects on a person's emotional state or thought processes.

regression: A return to an earlier stage of development; a mental mechanism used to resolve conflict by returning to a behavior that was more successful in having one's needs met.

schizophrenia: A severe and persistent mental illness characterized by disordered thinking, impaired social and vocational functioning; the most disabling of the mental illnesses.

somatic: Pertaining to the body; somatic signs and symptoms of emotional or mental disorders may include decreased appetite, insomnia, gastrointestinal distress, and decreased libido.

sleep paralysis: a temporary inability to talk or move when falling asleep or waking up, which may last a few seconds to minutes.

splitting: A defensive mechanism in which a person sees most objects as either good or bad and cannot distinguish the "gray," seeing only in "black or white"; the person often behaves in a manner that reinforces this way of viewing others and the world (e.g., a patient identifies a particular staff member as "the only one who truly understands me" and all others as "they don't care for me like you do," thereby working members of the staff against each other or "splitting" their cohesiveness and therefore their effectiveness in helping the person).

tangential speech: A pattern of speech in which a person strays from the subject at hand, going off into topics that have no relevance to the current discussion.

tardive dyskinesia: A movement disorder as an adverse effect of long-term use (at least 6 months) of antipsychotics (major tranquilizers); characterized by involuntary, choreathetoid movements of the upper extremities and facial muscles; may become severely disabling.

therapeutic relationships: Helping relationships between a patient and a mental health professional in which the "therapeutic use of self" principle is combined with the behavioral and psychosocial sciences to assist the patient on the road to recovery; these relationships falls within strict ethical boundaries.

thioxanthenes: A class of antipsychotic medications; includes chlorprothixene and thiothixene.

thought content: The subject focus of a person's thinking; in psychiatric assessments, thought content that is negativistic, fearful, lonely, suspicious, and so forth may be clues to emotional or mental disorders.

tolerance: The need for greatly increased amounts of the substance to achieve intoxication (or desired effect) or a markedly diminished effect with continued use of the same amount of the substance.

withdrawal: A maladaptive behavioral change, with physiological and cognitive concomitants, that occurs when blood or tissue concentrations of a substance decline in an individual who had maintained prolonged heavy use of the substance.

BIBLIOGRAPHY

American Foundation For Suicide Prevention. (AFFSP) (2003). Facts About Suicide. Retrieved from http://www.afsp.org/index-1.htm

Agency for Healthcare Research and Quality (AHRQ). (2002). Screening for Depression, What's New from the USPSTF. (Publication No. APPIP020019). Retrieved from http://www.ahrq.gov/clinic/uspstf/3rduspstf/depression/depresswh.htm

American Hospital Association. (1992). *A patient's bill of rights.* Chicago: American Hospital Association. Retrieved from http://www.cancer.org/docroot/MIT/content/MIT_3_2_Patients_Bill_Of_Rights.asp

American Nurses Association. (2001). *The Code of Ethics for Nurses.* Washington, DC. American Nurses Association. Retrieved from http://www.nursingworld.org/ethics/chcode.htm

American Nurses Association, American Psychiatric Nurses Association. (2000). *A statement on the scope and standards of psychiatric-mental health clinical nursing practice.* Washington, DC: American Nurses Association.

American Psychiatric Association. (2000). (*DSM-IV-TR*). *Diagnostic and statistical manual of mental disorders* (4th ed., text revision). Washington, DC: American Psychiatric Association.

Banos, J.H., & Franklin, L.M. (2002). Factor Structure of the Mini-Mental State Examination in Adult Psychiatric Inpatients. *Psychological Assessment, 14*(4):397-400.

Beck, A.T. (1967). *Depression: Clinical, experimental and theoretical aspects.* New York: Harper & Row.

Beck, A.T. (1976). *Cognitive therapy and the emotional disorders.* New York: International Universities Press.

Biers, Sam. (2003). Tarasoff v. Regents of the University of California S. Ct. of CA, 1976. Retrieved from http://www.4lawschool.com/torts/uc.htm

Citty, K.K., & Maynard, C.K. (1986). Managing manipulation. *Journal of Psychosocial Nursing, 24*:9-13.

Clemens-Stone, S., McGuire, S.L., & Eigsti, D.G. (2002). *Comprehensive community health nursing: Family, aggregate & community practice.* St. Louis, MO: Mosby.

Corcoran, D.K. (1988). Helping patients who've had near-death experiences. *Nursing 88, 11*:34-39.

Cowdry, R. (2001). *Major depression. The National Alliance for the Mentally Ill (NAMI).* Retrieved from http://www.nami.org/helpline/depress.htm

DiMatteo, M.R., Lepper, H.S., & Croghan, T.W. (2000). Depression is a risk factor for noncompliance with medical treatment meta-analysis of the effects of anxiety and depression on patient adherence. *Arch Intern Med, 160*:2101-2107.

Duke, L.M., Seltzer, B., Seltzer, J.E., & Vasterling, J.J. (2002). Cognitive components of deficit awareness in Alzheimer's disease. *Neuropsychology, 16*(3):359-369.

Flagg, M. (2001). Uvulopalatopharyngoplasty for sleep apnea. Retrieved from http://www.questdiagnostics.com/kbase/topic/detail/surgical/hw48958/detail.htm

Friedman, M., & Rosenman, R. (1974). *Type A behavior and your heart.* New York: Knopf.

Groves, J.E. (1978). Taking care of the hateful patient. *New England Journal of Medicine, 298,* 883-887.

Hussar, D.A. (2003). *The Merck manual of medical information – home edition. In compliance with drug treatment.* Retrieved from http://www.merck.com/pubs/mmanual_home2/sec02/ch016/ch016a.htm

Jaret, P. (2001). 10 Ways to improve patient compliance. *Hippocrates, 15*(2). Retrieved from http://www.hippocrates.com/FebruaryMarch2001/02features/02feat_compliance.html

Jacobs, J.W., Bernhard, M.R., Delgado, A., & Strain, J.J. (1977). Screening for organic mental syndrome in the medically ill. *Annuals of Internal Medicine, 86*:40-46.

Kaplan, H.I., & Sadock, B.J. (1991). Synopsis of psychiatry: *Behavioral Sciences Clinical Psychiatry* (6th ed.). Baltimore: Williams & Wilkins.

Kumler, F.R. (1963). The interpersonal interpretation of manipulation. In S.F. Burd & M.S. Marshall (Eds.), *Some clinical approaches to psychiatric nursing.* New York: Macmillan.

Laux, J.M. (2002). A primer on suicidology: Implications for counselors. *Journal of Counseling and Development, 80*(3):380-3.

Long, P.W. (2003). Internet Mental Health: Medications. Retrieved from http://www.mentalhealth.com/

Mayo Foundation for Medical Education and Research (MFMER). (2003). Depression (Signs and Symptoms). Retrieved from http://www.mayoclinic.com/invoke.cfm?objectid=F61D92BD-C12C-4C1E-98CE1DDC09196EA2

Mayo Foundation for Medical Education and Research (MFMER). (2002). Bipolar disorder. Retrieved from http://www.mayoclinic.com/invoke.cfm?id=DS00356

MEDLINEplus. (2003). Sleep Disorders. Retrieved from http://www.nlm.nih.gov/medlineplus/sleepdisorders.html

National Institute of Neurological Disorders and Stroke (NINDS). (2003). Brain Basics: Understanding Sleep. Retrieved from http://www.ninds.nih.gov/health_and_medical/pubs/understanding_sleep_brain_basic_.htm

National Institute of Neurological Disorders and Stroke (NINDS). (2001). NINDS Narcolepsy Information Page. Retrieved from http://www.ninds.nih.gov/health_and_medical/disorders/narcolep_doc.htm

National Institute for Occupational Safety and Health (NIOSH). (2002). Violence: Occupational Hazards in Hospitals DHHS (NIOSH) Publication No. 2002–101. Retrieved from http://www.cdc.gov/niosh/2002-101.html

North American Nursing Diagnosis Association. (2003). *Nursing diagnoses: Definitions & classification, 2003-2004.* Philadelphia: NANDA.

Peplau, H.E. (1952). *Interpersonal relations in nursing.* New York: Putnam.

Sanchez, H.G. (2001). Risk factor model for suicide assessment and intervention. *Professional Psychology — Research & Practice, 32*(4): 351-358.

Schroy, P.C. (2002). Barriers to colorectal cancer screening: Part 1 — patient noncompliance. *General Medicine, 4*(2). Retrieved from http://www.medscape.com/viewarticle/432891

Selye, H. (1976). *The stress of life* (rev. ed.). New York: McGraw-Hill.

Spratto, G.R., & Woods, A.L. (2003). *PDR nurse's drug handbook.* Retrieved from http://www.nursespdr.com/

Sternbach, H. (2003). Serotonin syndrome: How to avoid, identify, & treat dangerous drug interactions. *Current Psychiatry Online, 2*(5). Retrieved from http://www.currentpsychiatry.com/2003_05/0503_serotonin.asp

Stuart, G.W. (2002). *Pocket guide to psychiatric nursing.* (5th ed.). St. Louis, MO: Mosby.

Thobaben, M. (2000). "…About suicide". *Nursing 2000, 30*(10):73, October 2000.

Thobaben, M. (2002). The aftermath of the terrorists attack on September 11, 2001: Post-traumatic stress disorder. *Home Health Care Management & Practice, 14*:5, 398-399.

Thobaben, M. (2003). *Ethical principles and clinical practice.* Class Notes.

Thobaben, M. (2000). Improving client compliance with taking antidepressant medication. *Home Care Provider, 6*(1):8-9.

Thobaben, M. (2001). Strategies to overcome insomnia. *Home Care Provider, 6*(2):46-47.

Thobaben, M. (2002). Screening for depression: ask clients two simple questions. *Home Health Care Management & Practice, 15*(1):82-83.

U.S. Department of Health & Human Services. (2003). Protecting the Privacy of Patients' Health Information. Retrieved from http://www.hhs.gov/news/facts/privacy.html

U.S. Department of Health & Human Services. Centers for Disease Control and Prevention (CDC). (2003). Suicide in the United States. Retrieved from http://www.cdc.gov/ncipc/factsheets/suifacts.htm

U.S. Department of Health and Human Services. National Institute of Mental Health (NIMH). (2003). Breaking Ground, Breaking Through: The Strategic Plan for Mood Disorders Research. Retrieved from http://www.nimh.nih.gov/strategic/stplan_mooddisorders.cfm

U.S. Department of Labor: Occupational Safety & Health Administration (OSHA). (2003). OSH Act of 1970. Retrieved from http://www.osha.gov/pls/oshaweb/owasrch.search_form?p_doc_type=OSHACT&p_toc_level=0&p_keyvalue=

Wiley, P.L. (1968). Manipulation. In L.T. Zderad & H.C. Belcher (Eds.), *Developing behavioral concepts in nursing.*

World Fellowship For Schizophrenia And Allied Disorders (WFFSAAD). (2003). Schizophrenia: The Myths, the Signs, The Statistics. Retrieved from http://www.world-schizophrenia.org/publications/18-myths.html

Note: All on-line research was completed September–November, 2003.

INDEX

O

P

S

T

U

V

W

Z

PRETEST KEY

Psychiatric Principles and Applications for General Patient Care

1.	c	Chapter 1
2.	d	Chapter 1
3.	a	Chapter 2
4.	d	Chapter 3
5.	c	Chapter 4
6.	b	Chapter 5
7.	c	Chapter 6
8.	a	Chapter 7
9.	c	Chapter 8
10.	b	Chapter 9
11.	d	Chapter 9
12.	a	Chapter 10
13.	b	Chapter 10
14.	d	Chapter 11
15.	b	Chapter 12
16.	a	Chapter 13
17.	a	Chapter 14
18.	c	Chapter 14
19.	c	Chapter 15
20.	b	Chapter 16

Notes

Notes

Notes

Notes

Notes